Poor man's way to fight cancer

by Peter Rogers MD, copyright July 2023

You are fat and sick, because you eat the wrong food, and yo   . That's good, because it means you can fix it.

Subtitle: Cancer Picture Book

In the name of the Starch, the Fruit & the Vegetable, let us pray. The **TEN COMMANDMENTS** of nutrition are written in stone. Follow them & you will be born again into better bodyweight & better health.

1. **Starch is the true god of food.**

   - Thou shalt put no other foods before starch.
   - Starches include **potatos**, sweet potatos, rice, beans, oatmeal, quinoa, millet, carrots.
   - Eat starch to satisfy hunger, and to provide energy.
   - Starch is the Way. Starch is the Entree.
   - Starch should provide 60-90% of your calories.

2. **Thine brain is a thermostat.**

   - Hypothalamic hunger center forces you to eat exactly the amount of food that you do.
   - Hunger is set by all mighty, hunger drive, & it will crush any willpower attempts to change.
   - "Eat less and exercise more" is the mantra of chumps. It does not work.
   - The thermostat can **only be re-set by changing** what you eat.
   - You do not need to count calories.
   - Eat the right foods, and the body will correctly program itself.

3. **Vegetables are the best source of nutrients**.

   - Fruits are good in limited amounts.
   - If thou art young, and skinny, or if thou exerciseth much, then thou may eatheth more fruit.
   - For every meal thou must ask thyself three questions.
     1. **What starch?**
     2. **What vegetable?**
     3. **What fruit?**

4. **Plants provide what you need to spread your seed.**

   - Plant foods optimize your sex appeal.
   - Vegetables vasodilate by increasing nitric oxide, potassium, and magnesium.
   - Better blood flow gives you the glow of vitality.

5. **It's not a diet! It's a Way of life.**

6. **Thou shalt not eat meat.**

   - Meat makes you fat. Milk is liquid meat.
   - Cheese is meat jello; when you eat it, you look like the animal it came from.
   - Pizza looks same on your plate, and in your arteries; like atherosclerosis plaques.
   - Meat causes leaky gut, xenosialitis, inflammation, and autoimmune disease.
   - Meat causes constipation, abdominal pressure syndrome.
   - Meat causes iron overload, estrogen overload, and **tumor promotion.**

7. **Thou shalt not eat oils.**

   - Oils are liquid fat, and make you fat.
   - Oils are **tumor promoters.**
   - If you must go to a restaurant, then choose the buffet, and eat your salad without dressing.
   - Skip the dressing and you will look better undressed.
   - Salad dressing is for pussies. Sodium is for dummies (causes hypertension).

8. **Thou shalt not commit adultery with junk food, and fast food.**

9. **Thou shalt not bear false witness against the vegan diet.**

   - There are two kingdoms of food.
   - The vegan kingdom is the land of healthy aging like the Tarahumara, Okinawa, Yanomamo, rural Kenya, Sardinia, and Loma Linda.
   - The meat-junk food kingdom is the land of the fat & sick, like Pima & most Americans.
   - You may ask, "What about fat vegans?"
     - They have fallen into temptation of oils and sweets: the siren song of "philosophic" vegetarians.
     - Do not be fooled by those false prophets.
   - The path to optimal body weight is **ORTHODOX VEGANISM,** low sodium, low fat, whole food, 100% organic, 100% vegan, starch based, with no oil-caffeine-alcohol-sweets.
   - Does that sound like too much effort? Get thee an **ATTITUDE OF GRATITUDE**. Heel your objections to Veganism, and it may heal you.
   - When the rest of your age cohort is fat, diabetic, woodless, hooked on hypertension pills, mentally slow, and worried about open heart surgery;
   - you will be waking up with wood, and the only question will be whether to bop the bishop, or bang the Betty. Starch has saved you.

10. **Thou shalt not covet thy neighbor's plate.**

    - of G-M-O fed, hormonally hypertrophied, antibiotic assaulted, hexane extracted, MSG marinated, trans fat fried, Frankenstein food.

Welcome to Health Purgatory:

Restore hope all ye who enter.

"In middle age, I found myself in a dark wood, and the path was lost." - Dante from "the Divine Comedy."

You can make it to Health Paradise.

Theme song:

Winners eat starch and fruits,
for six pack abs,
and a horn that toots.

Thesis:

Become a vegan or you're f_cked for health.

Plant eaters are healthier, because that is what we are made to eat; premium fuel for premium performance.

Motto:

Vegan today. Vegan tomorrow. Vegan forever!!

Table of contents

Dedication:

To my dear wife Effy. Eff you I love. You are the mother effer of our children. Sometimes I do wish you would eff off.

Disclaimer:

"I have nothing to declare but my genius" – Oscar Wilde.

This book is for educational purposes only. It is NOT medical advice. I am not your doctor.

I'm just a lonely, old, autistic hermit who writes these books, because I have nothing else to do.

Dietary change can have a powerful effect on blood pressure and blood glucose.

If you are taking any medications, you should let your doctor know, before changing your diet, as you will likely need to change medication dosages.

Chapter #1 **Boreword:**

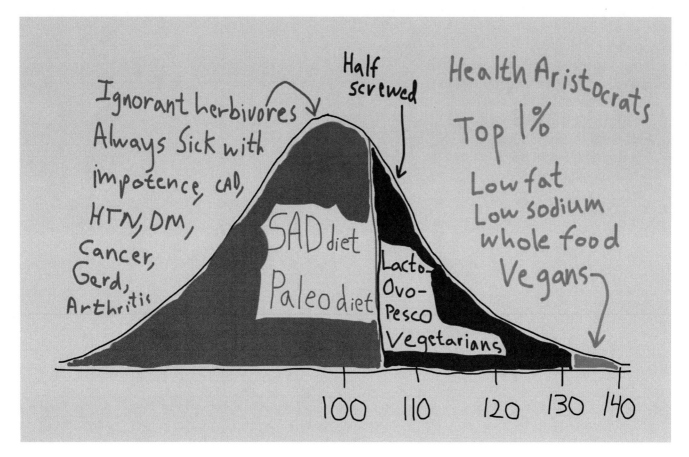

Figure #1: **Normal distribution** drawing shows that only about 1% of people have even a moderate understanding of nutrition. Learning what to eat is easy. The hard part is unlearning all the nonsense promulgated by popular culture.

What's new in this book = drawings! With my earlier books, I didn't know how to draw on a computer. I've also learned more about cancer pathophysiology & treatments since the last book, "Journey to optimal health."

The way to get the most out of this book is to **look at the pictures; then read it; then watch the internet videos by me on cancer & related topics.**

Then watch more videos on cancer by Dr John McDougall, T. Colin Campbell Phd, Ruth Heidrich Phd, etc.

Key points:

You can do a lot to reduce your risk of cancer.
Cancer patients can do a lot to improve their chance of long term survival.
The somatic mutation theory (SMT) has been largely refuted.
The metabolic theory of cancer (MTC) explains cancer causation, and how to prevent it. The MTC gives you logical strategies to try to slow cancer growth.

My videos are mostly at You Tube channel "Peter Rogers MD." I also have videos at bitchute dot com & rumble dot com, twitter dot com & linked in dot com. If you tube ever gives me the boot, I will move everything to bitchute & rumble, and to other internet video sites.

In the book "Mystery Method" by Mystery, about seducing women, he described the average guy as an AFC = Average Frustrated Chump. In this book I will describe the average person as an ADS = Average Dumb Shit. We will call the Wise Patient a WP.

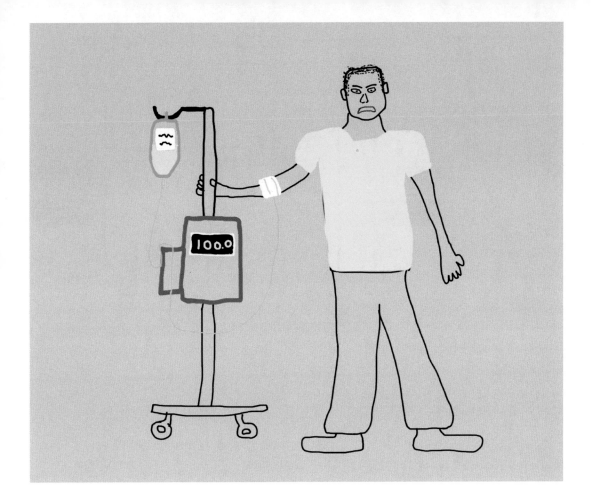

Fig #2: **Chemotherapy patient**.

"To just go for surgery & chemo is easy. You just sign the consent form. That's **passive**.
To study cancer, & completely change your diet, your exercise, your habits, your attitude towards life.

That's difficult. That takes a lot of effort. That's active"
– Chris Wark, long term survivor of colon cancer & author of "Chris beat cancer"

I like Chris Wark, and he has good things to say, especially about the psychology of recovering from cancer.
I disagree with his advice on olive oil. I recommend to avoid all oils. Oils are highly processed liquid fat.

The typical ADS (Average Dumb Shit) is all emotional when they walk into a cancer doctor office. ADS
says, "I want this cancer gone. Can you cut it out with surgery? Yes, of course I'll take chemo."

Famous last words.

The WP (Wise Person) knows that the cancer has probably been there at least a decade. They know they've
got some time to study. Chemo only works well for a few cancers like some leukemias, lymphomas,
testicular cancer, small cell lung cancer, etc.

The attitude in conventional medicine is often that, "The patient is going to die anyways, so we might as
well try chemo."

Unless chemo was proven to generate a BIG improvement in survival, eg. > 30%, then I would NOT take it.
It's pretty much guaranteed to cause unpleasant side effects.

In the past, whenever I saw a chemo patient with a bald head, I used to immediately feel sorry for them.

Now, I say to myself, probably an ADS, who was too lazy to read about their disease.

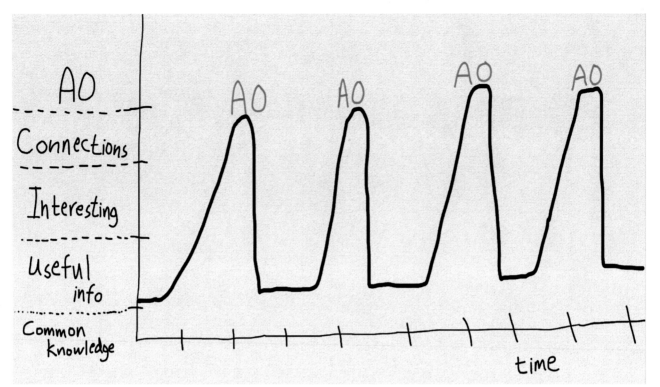

Fig 3: Multiple **AO (Academic Orgasm)** approach to public speaking. I promise to go slow and be gentle!

The **useful info** in the drawing above is stuff you need to know = **general understanding of cancer**. The next step up is **interesting info** = **a little more technical**. The "connections" are explanations of how relates to other topics in health & nutrition. **AO"s are Academic Orgasms.**

The point is that this book will at times leap into the stratosphere of transcedent understanding, but will always soon return to the practical aspects of staying healthy.

I usually will only have one illustration per page, because this word processor program is kind of fussy with images, and torments me with crazy behavior if I try to put two images on the same page.

Kind of like a crazy girlfriend who senses you'll put up with her games, because she knows you don't have any other good options.

Rule #1 of preventing cancer (& of trying to slow cancer growth) is NO MEAT! From now on, when I say "preventing cancer" it will also mean "trying to slow cancer growth."

The same things that prevent cancer are almost always potentially helpful for trying to slow cancer growth. I have to speak a little euphemistically about all this diet & lifestyle stuff, because big pharma has billions of dollars & they don't like doctors educating the proles.

For what it's worth, I live the anti-cancer lifestyle to the max, and do all the stuff I'm recommending for you in terms of optimizing diet, and avoiding toxins.

I'm proud of that fact that I'm aging better than all the people I know at my age, 59 years old, and especially than my wife.

In our younger days, we went to a party, and she said to me, "Do you know what people think when they see us?" I could tell she was up to no good, but I played along. "What?"

She said, "What is such a beautiful woman, doing with such an ugly man?" I said, "I thought they were thinking, what's such a smart man doing with such a stupid woman?"

Now that I'm the better looking one, I could've taken advantage of the situation by sleeping with her friends; but I didn't; because I don't want to ruin those friendships for her; because she likes to visit them; it gets her out of the house; so I can have some peace and quiet.

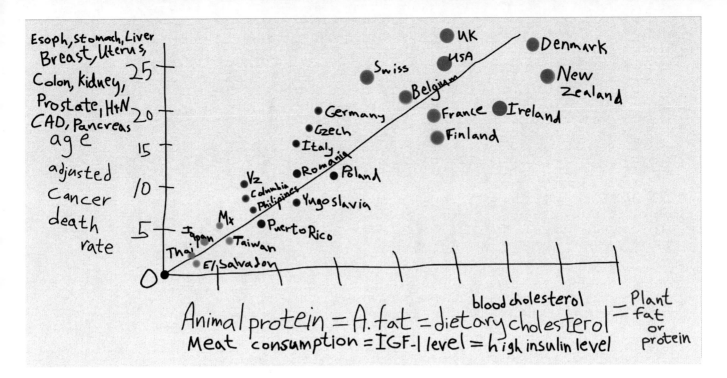

Fig 4: **Graph of cancer & western diseases vs dietary animal protein** = saturated fat = dietary cholesterol = meat consumption = IGF level = insulin level. They all generate the same relationship, because they're all related. Idea for this graph comes from the work of T Colin Campbell Phd (TCC) in his research papers, his books & his online lectures. TCC figured out that the more animal protein eaten, the more cancer.

Animal food is just animal protein + animal fat (mostly **saturated fat**). That's why saturated fat intake is a good approximation of animal protein intake.

Animal food does not have any carbohydrate (except for milk). Animal food has ZERO fiber.

All mammal cells stabilize their plasma membranes with cholesterol, so all animal food has **cholesterol**. That's why dietary cholesterol is a good approximation of animal protein intake.

Animal protein has an anabolic effect on the human body that raises blood cholesterol. That's one of the reasons why elevated blood cholesterol is an approximation of animal protein intake.

Elevated blood cholesterol also causes atherosclerosis; and atherosclerosis increases risk of tissue hypoxia [oxygen deficit]; and hypoxia can cause cancer.

Animal protein causes activation of mTOR. MTOR is a nutrient sensing pathway, that is like a building contractor getting ready to build a building. The contractor cannot build until he has all the building materials available. To build means to enable the cell to replicate. A cell has to double its contents of DNA, RNA, proteins & membranes before it can replicate. The rate limiting step is often the availability of leucine and methionine.

Animal protein has more leucine & methionine (compared with plant protein). So animal protein causes activation of mTOR. Cancer patients do NOT want activation of mTOR. If a cancer patient can block mTOR, they can slow down the growth of cancer.

Preventing mTOR activation is like **the Fabian strategy** that the ancient Romans used against Hannibal. Hannibal the Carthaginian general kicked the crap out of the Romans in several open battles, killing tens of thousands of Romans. The Romans were quite afraid of Hannibal.

Then Fabius Quintus Maximus stepped forward and said he had figured out how to defeat Hannibal. Fabius said, "Hannibal is far from Carthage. His supply lines are weak. If we can deprive his army of food, they will shrink, and retreat."

Fabius & the Romans won the victory by starving Hannibal into retreat.

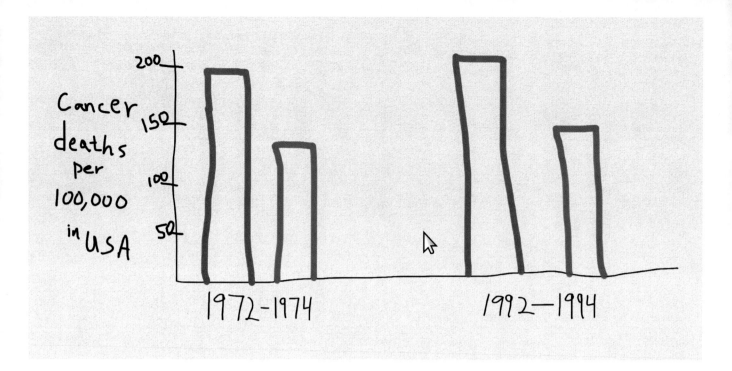

Fig 5: **Cancer deaths over time.** Red = men, pink = women. Key point is that there has been almost ZERO progress since 1972 when "war on cancer" was declared for the chemo approach. The point is that chemo has not improved much since 1972.

Yes, of course, the chemo companies keep trotting out new drugs, but the drugs don't do much. Chemo gets overhyped, because it's SUPER PROFITABLE. The drug companies have ZERO incentive to look for other approaches.

ADS thinks that universities and corporations are hard at work doing research, and trying to figure out how to save him. **Chemo companies & hospitals know that they get their money whether the patient lives of dies.**

One of the dirty little secrets about modern medicine is that it's atheistic, and does not care much about patients. **Conventional medicine defines a "standard of care" for treatment of diseases. The standard is always made for low functioning people.**

It has to be for low functioning people, because the majority of patients are low functioning eg. alcoholics, tobacco smokers, drug addicts, functional illiterates, cognitively slow diabetics, low IQ dummies, etc.

The problem is that the "standard of care" is what's offered to all patients. **High functioning people should want more than the standard of care. They should want OPTIMAL CARE!**

The reason optimal care is not routinely suggested is because it usually depends on the patient. The patient has to learn about nutrition, toxicology, stress management, exercise, sleep, etc.

ADS can't do this. They don't have the intellectual curiosity or literacy to learn much.

That's why the patient must do a lot of studying on their own. One of the reasons that doctors tend to begin conversations with a polite, professional, dopey tone is because they are so used to talking to cognitively slow patients.

One of my internal medicine friends told me that almost all of her over 60 years old patients were cognitively impaired. Another told me that most of his patients over 50 were mentally slow. My psychiatrist friend told me that most of his psychiatry patients didn't just have psychiatric diseases, they were usually stupid.

The point is that **if a person is willing to study & learn, they have a good chance to be MUCH HEALTHIER than ADS's.**

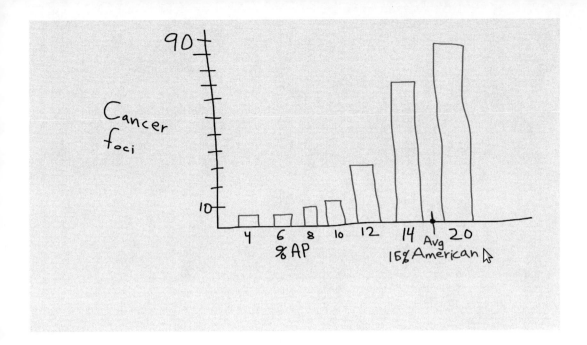

Fig 6: **Number of cancer foci in rodents in comparison with percent (%) of calories from animal protein (AP).** This graph is based on the research of T Colin Campbell which was discussed in his research papers and his masterpiece book "China Study," and his many online lectures. TCC wrote other good books like "Whole" & "Future of nutrition."

TCC says Americans were eating 15% protein, but I think it's higher than that. Americans tend to eat lots of animal protein.

T Colin Campbell (TCC) deserves a Nobel prize for figuring out that animal protein causes cancer. They will never give him the Nobel prize, because they don't want the public to know that animal protein has such a strong effect towards causing cancer.

TCC showed that the more animal protein the rodents got, the more cancer they got. TCC showed that if he stopped giving the rodents animal protein, that the cancers stopped growing!

That's an important point.

TCC showed that if he removed animal protein from the rodent diet, their cancers stopped growing!

TCC was so confident in the results of his research, because he did his experiments in multiple variations, and however he looked at it, **animal protein was THE MAJOR cause of cancer.**

TCC was so confident of his research, that when his wife was diagnosed with melanoma, a type of cancer, he had her go on a vegan diet, and she did great!

TCC said **there is no safe lower level of animal protein consumption; it's best & safest to not eat any animal protein.**

TCC said, "Animal protein is the most important cause of cancer."

A good way to think of it is that animal protein is the most important PROMOTER of cancer growth.

To summarize:

WP's know that the best diet has ZERO animal protein. No meat, not one bite!

This includes dairy. No milk, not one drop!

Same goes for any dairy product like cheese or yoghurt. I would NEVER eat these foods.

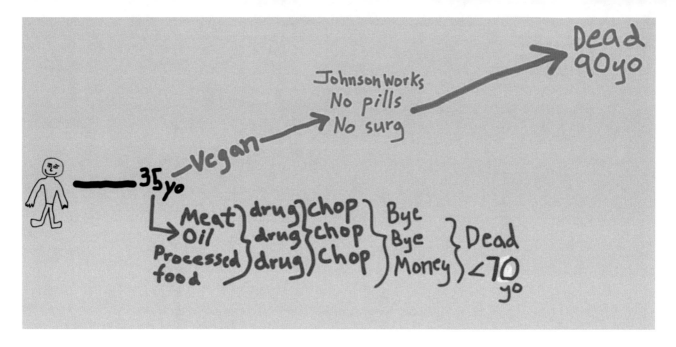

Fig 7: **To be or not to be a low fat vegan.** This is your choice. It's your life. You either do the healthy stuff like low fat, low sodium vegan, and exercise, or you end up an ADS (Average DumbShit).

ADS get fat and sick by 30's or 40's, and end up multiple pills, before they get sent for surgery. Pills and surgery sometimes slow things down a little bit, but WP's (Wise Persons) can do better.

WP's can usually live much longer, and much healthier.

"If you feed a herbivore a high fat diet, they all develop atherosclerosis, 100%." - William C. Roberts MD (best cardiac pathologist in the world).

Humans are herbivores. If you feed them a high fat diet, they all develop atherosclerosis.

Atherosclerosis blocks arteries. Atherosclerosis decreases oxygen delivery to tissues. **Lack of oxygen is called "hypoxia."**

Mild hypoxia tends to cause cell dysfunction = decreased cell productivity.

Severe hypoxia causes cells to die suddenly. Sudden death of a cell is called "necrosis."

Moderate hypoxia usually causes cells to die gradually. Gradual cell death is called **"apoptosis."** Apoptosis enables a cell to recycle itself. Recycling means that the proteins another cell components can be packaged into vesicles and used by other cells.

Moderate hypoxia prevents the cell from using its mitochondria for oxygen related production of ATP (Adenosine TriPhosphate). Moderate hypoxia can also cause a cell to transform into a cancer cell.

When a human cell is transformed into a cancer cell, it tends to behave very much like an anaerobic bacteria.

Hypoxia induced transformation of a normal human cell into a cancer cell is called the **Warburg effect.**

The Warburg effect is one of the keys to understanding cancer.

	Sat fat	Oil	Sodium	Tob	Fruits & vegetables	Dm	Htn	MI	Stroke	Impotence	Cancer
American	High	mod	Moderate 6 g/d	Low	Low	Mod to high	Mod to High	High	Moderate	High	High
E. Asian, Japan, Korea, China	Low	Low	High > 12 g/d	High	Moderate	Low	High	Low	High		Moderate
S. Asian, India	Low to mod (dairy)	High	High	Low	Low	High	High	High	mod	High	
Low fat, low sodium, vegan	Low	ZERO	Low	ZERO	High	Very Low	Very Low	ZERO	Very low	Very low	Very low

Fig 8: **SAD = Standard American Diet** = leads to high risk of heart disease and cancer. East Asian diet, like old Japan is a big improvement, but too much sodium. India common diet has too much fried food, and too much dairy. **The low fat, low sodium, whole food, 100% vegan, 100% organic is the best diet by far**; it lowers the risk of all the common diseases.

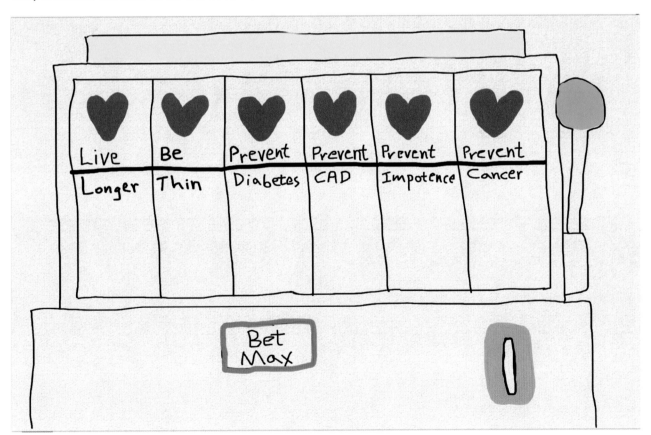

Fig 9: Low fat, low sodium, whole food, 100% vegan, 100% organic is your best chance for winning the jackpot for health.

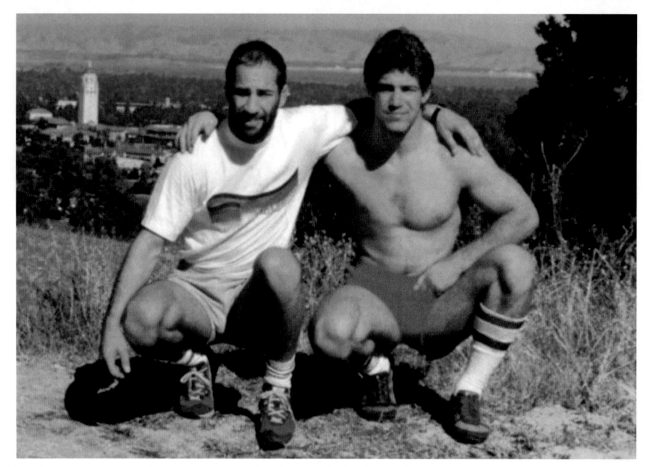

Fig 10: **Dave Schultz incrementalism & Mark Schultz intensity of purpose** against cancer.

Photo shows Dave & Mark Schultz at Stanford, on one of the training hills for Stanford team to run sprints. Freshman year at Stanford, the wrestling team ran sprints on the hills, and I noticed that Dave was slow.

In the weight room, he was weak. He was also fat compared to other wrestlers. I wondered, how did a fat, weak & slow guy become national champion?

When he was a kid, he was fat and dyslexic. His nickname was "Pudge." He got called names like "fat dumbass."

He liked wrestling and sought out the best coaching. In junior high he trained with the Palo Alto high school team, and the Stanford university team. His secret was to focus on wrestling technique in an incremental way, to learn everything about technique.

How do you win, when you have no money?

How do you win, when you don't have much talent?

Here's the secret:

Willingness to learn is a great talent.

Learning a bunch of small skills, can add up to be a great talent

You can learn everything about cancer prevention.

You can do a whole bunch of things that might add up to a big benefit. I'm not allowed to say "will" add up to a big benefit, but I can assure you that I do all these things, and they have provided a big benefit to me, and to many people who have done the same.

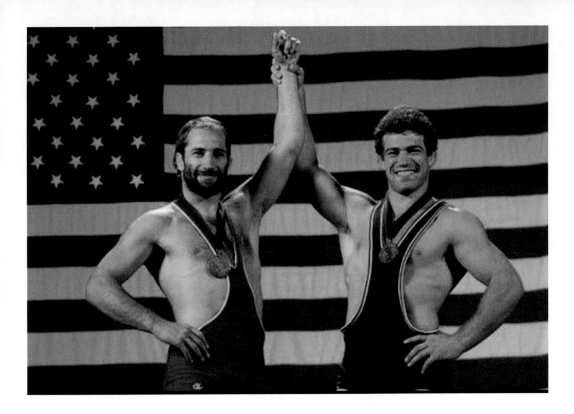

Fig 11: **Dave Schultz incrementalism** = to learn every detail of technique in his sport → you can only increase strength & conditioning about 20% (analog)

→ you can increase technique 1,000% (logarithmic) → he studied technique of all the best wrestlers in the world → he taught himself to speak Russian so

he could learn their technique → he was best technical wrestler in the world

Mark Schultz intensity of purpose = to focus all your energy on the goal
→ "the only thing I care about right now, is wrestling = (the year he won his first world championship) → The only thing I own is this motorcycle, and it's a piece of crap." - Mark Schultz.

I had a recurrent shoulder injury, and the head coach thought he was wasting a scholarship on me. I told a friend that I was thinking of quitting, and he told Mark Schultz.

Mark said to me, "Pete, you shouldn't quit. You train with me. On Tuesdays & Thursdays we will run stadium stairs.

You need to hang around with wrestlers. The guys who are serious about wrestling should all live in an athlete fraternity. You guys should be talking about wrestling. You need to focus your energy on wrestling. You will improve.

Your opponent is your worst enemy in the world. He is trying to beat you up, and embarrass you in front of your friends.
You should devote every ounce of energy that you have to fighting him.

The next year, I became team captain, and set the all time Stanford university record of 39 wins in one season & won student athlete of year award.

If you use these methods of incrementalism & intensity of purpose, you might make much more progress than you previously imagined.

I promise to get to all the cancer pathophysiology in a moment, but this backstory of wrestling and academics shows how this approach can make a giant improvement.

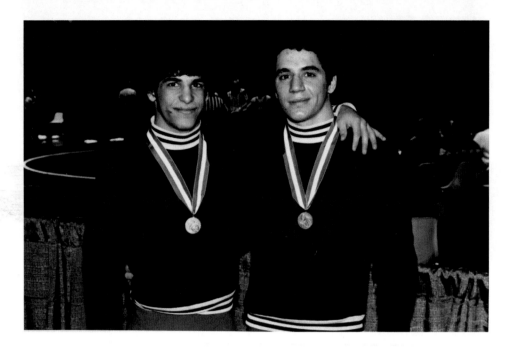

Fig 12: **Junior year high school,** my training partner, Senior John Giura won 1ˢᵗ place in state. As a junior I took 3ʳᵈ place with a 39-1 record. I was sad, because I should have won.

In a Spring, freestyle tournament, I fractured the growthplate of my clavicle (collarbone) and kept reinjuring it; and was unable to wrestle in the senior year state tournament. This was psyologically devastating for me.

The big wrestling schools lost interest in me, but Stanford still offered me a scholarship. That's how I ended up there. California seemed like a million miles away from Chicago.

In Chicago, I had a great family, a great home, great friends, and a great girlfriend. I was runner up for homecoming King at a high school with 1,100 students in each class. If I had been able to wrestle, I would have been homecoming King.

That's how much fun my life was, before I got sent to the college equivalent of "Siberia" known as Stanford. The loneliest college in the USA for athletes, especially wrestlers.

Some may say, well what about Harvard? No comparison. Harvard is in Boston = lots of young people around.

Stanford is in the middle of a cow pasture. There is no town. There's no young people, other than Stanford students who study all the time.

Star high school athletes are like celebrities at their high schools. At Stanford, even the guys that were going to go Pro in football and baseball, often weren't able to find a girfriend.

Guys at state schools have bars on campus that are open 6 nights a week, and parties every weekend. These guys told me all these stories. Their colleges were like social paradise compared with Stanford.

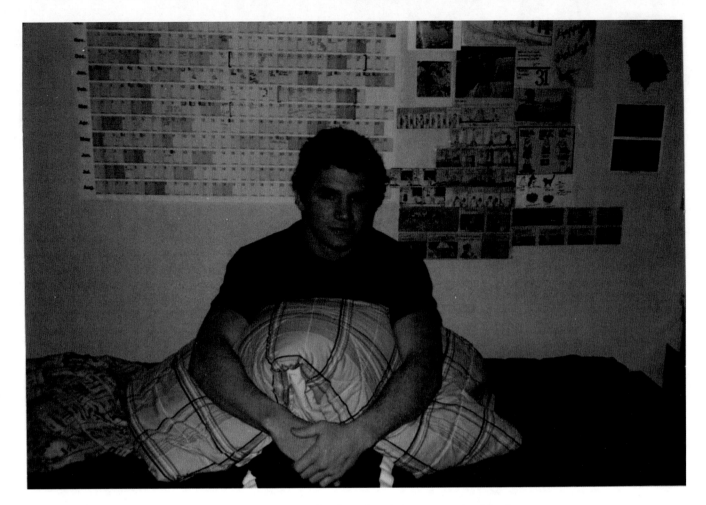

Fig 13: **The pathetic, lonely freshman at Stanford** with a Linus security blanket.

Calendar on the wall, counting the days until can go home, and see girlfriend.

I hated being so lonely; but it gave me a lot of time
to study the process of learning & memorizing large amounts of information.

Injuries had messed up my athletic career, but the lessons from Dave & Mark Schultz:

Intensity of purpose: be obsessed with improving in your field.

Incrementalism = be obsessed about learning every minute detail of your field & related topics,

These two methods showed me how to excel in academics.

I had screwed up my athletic career by trying to return to competition too soon.

I was not going to let anything screw up my academic career.

I was quite happy to study all day.

I would have loved to have a girlfriend at Stanford, but I was not going to let the lack of a girlfriend or anything else effect my attitude towards becoming a great scholar.

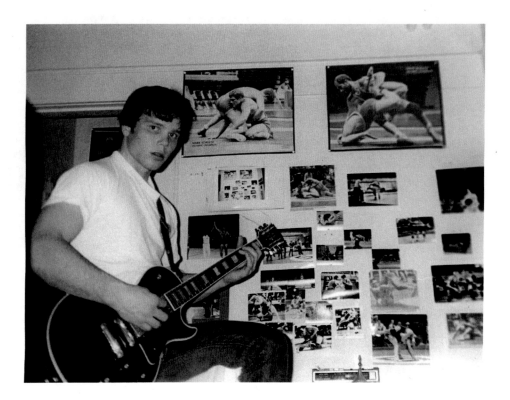

Fig 14: **Wall of fame in the athlete fraternity.** Olympic champion Schultz brothers on top. Then All Americans like Dave Lee. Dave Lee is the Rock & Roll wrestler, All American, National champion. My training partner.

Then guys like me, team captain. I set the record for most victories ever in a season at Stanford, because I was always fighting my way through wrestle backs to take 3rd or 5th in a tournament, and end up something like 6-2. Dave would just go 4-0, so I ended up with the most wins.

My training partners were All Americans, national champions and Olympic champions; so I was used to getting beat up every day in practice.

I was sad about being the low man on the totem pole, in the world of wrestling. I compensated by trying to become a great student. The Dabrowski & Adler concepts were helpful.

Dabrowski theory of personality disintegration & reintegration = you take your frustration about failing in one area, and use it to energize you in a new field of endeavor.

Alfred Adler inferiority principle = after failing in one area = one can take the energy of frustration & rechannel it into another area for success.

I was determined to become a great doctor or scientist; and **really wanted to learn,** not just get grades.

Sophomore year I got A pluses in the most difficult classes at Stanford like the weed out classes of organic chemistry & evolutionary biology.

The "average" student in the class was about 99.9% academically.

Once I knew that I could dominate that group academically, I knew I could dominate anything academic.

That's the benefit of incrementalism & intensity of purpose = the poor man's way used for academics.

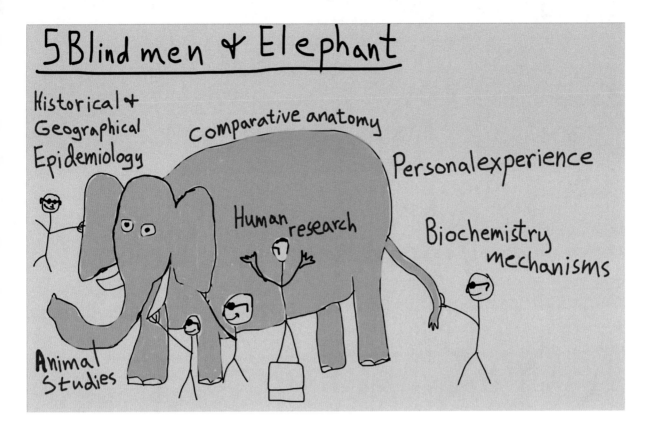

Fig 15: **5 blind men & an elephant**

#1 man at tail "it's a rope," #2 at leg "tree," #3 at tusk "spear," #4 at ear "rug," #5 at side "wall"

Listen to all viewpoints with an open mind.

Try to see the big picture; to have a bird's eye view.

Lesson: Learn the metabolic theory of cancer, and all the ways that you can improve the situation, and you might improve your health a lot.

"The first step to an intelligent conversation, is to remove emotions." - Aristotle

Typical patient gets all emotional. I've got cancer! I don't want this! Cut it out! I want surgery!

Smart patient studies their disease to learn all their options.

Typical patient rushes into surgery or chemotherapy, without ever studying their disease, and their options.

They often suffer, and even die from complications of chemo or surgery that they did NOT even need.

In the medical world, the price for being an ignoramus is very high, and often painful and fatal.

Smart patients make the most of diet & lifestyle options which are a much bigger topic than most doctors realize.

Look up Ruth Heidrich Phd, Janet Murray Wakelin, Chris Wark, Lorraine Day & many other vegans who exercise & studied stress management & are often very religious.   How are they doing?

The longest lived populations in the world are all religious. Religion unites people. Re-Ligion comes from Re-Ligare = to ligate = to tie together = social connections. People with social connections have lower stress, help each other, enjoy each others company, live longer.

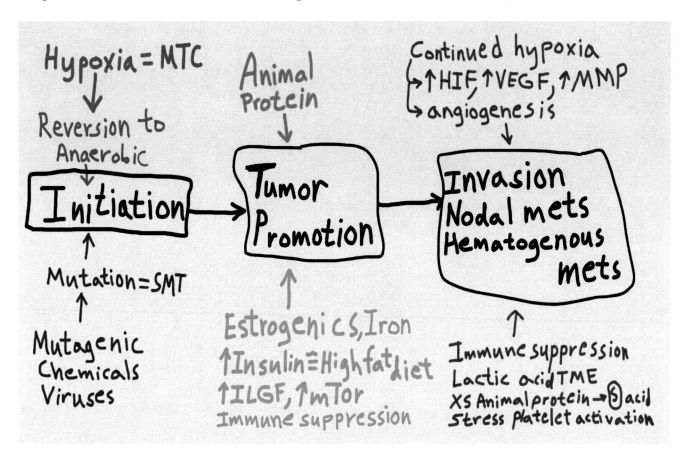

Fig 16: **The 3 stages of cancer.** Initiation = damage to DNA (usually causes bypoxia, but can be caused by toxic chemicals, etc). Then promotion = something that makes the tumor grow. Then invasion = where tumor spreads to other locations; via the blood (hematogeneous mets) or lymphatics or by direct growth into local tissues.

Everyone has some cells with DNA damage. This could have happened to you decades ago.

The promotion phase is where a person has the best chance to stop cancer growth.

1st you learn what makes cancer grows.

Then stop doing those things!!

Common tumor promoters include animal protein = meat and dairy;

Many high fat foods like vegetable oils are tumor promoters.

Excess dietary salt = sodium chloride = Na+Cl- = tumor promoter.

Estrogenic chemicals are cancer promoters = carcinogenic and obesity causers = obesogenic.

Immunosuppressants are tumor promoters.

You need your immune system to remove cancer cells.

Cortisol suppresses the immune system.

Psychological stress, sleep deprivation, and caffeine cause increased cortisol.

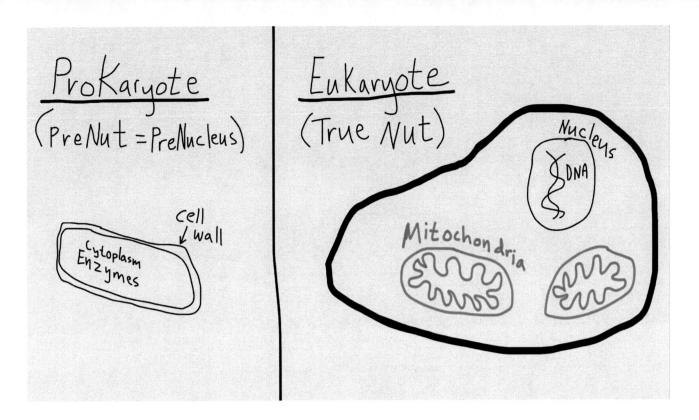

Fig 17: **Bacteria (ProKaryote) and human (EuKaryote) cells.** Pro means "before." Karyo means "nut or nucleus." Prokaryote = bacterial cell = cell with no nucleus.

Eu means true. Eu-Karyote = cell with a true nucleus. In reality, the most important feature of EuKaryotes is that they have mitochondria.

Mitochondria are the energy factories of a cell. The vast majority of cell energy in humans is made in mitochondria.

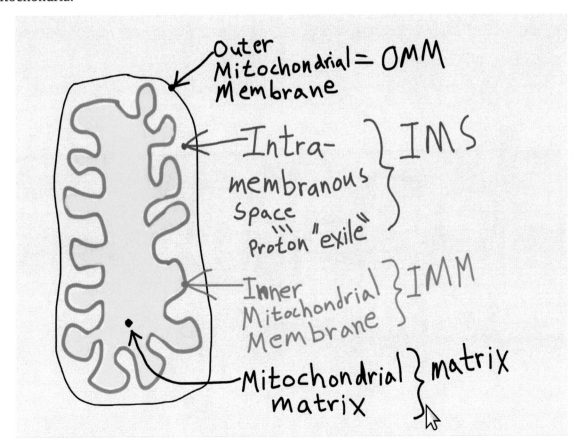

Fig 18: **Mitochondria parts: OMM** = Outer Mitochondrial Membrane. **IMS** = Inner Mitochondrial Membrane = the "container" for storing protons under pressure. **IMM** = Inner Mitochondrial Membrane = location for electron transfer chain proteins. **Matrix** = center of the mitochondria = location of Kreb's cycle = TriCarboxylic Acid (TCA) cycle = Citric acid cycle.

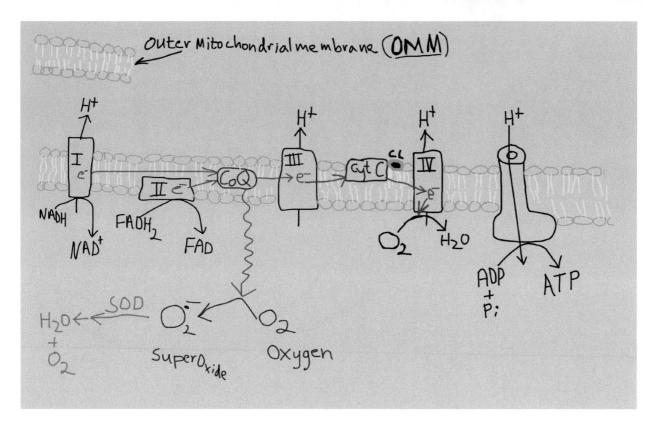

Fig 19: **Normal IMM and Electron Transport Chain (ETC).** Complexes 1, 2, 3, are like a fireman bucket brigade. Instead of passing along buckets, they pass along electrons. The final acceptor of the electrons is water = the "ultimate" electron acceptor.

Oxygen has the the second highest electronegativity (pulling power to attract electrons) of any element in the periodic table. So oxygen REALLY wants those electrons. The energy of electron transfer in complexes 1, 3, 4 is coupled to pumping protons from the mitochondrial matrix into the intramembranous space.

Normal mitochondrial electron transport & oxidative phosphorylation

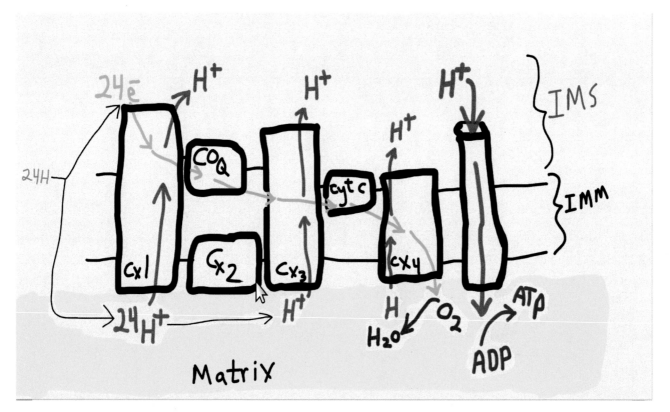

Fig 20: **Electron Transport Chain (ETC)** shows how electron transport is coupled to pumping protons from the matrix to the IMS (IntraMembranous Space),.

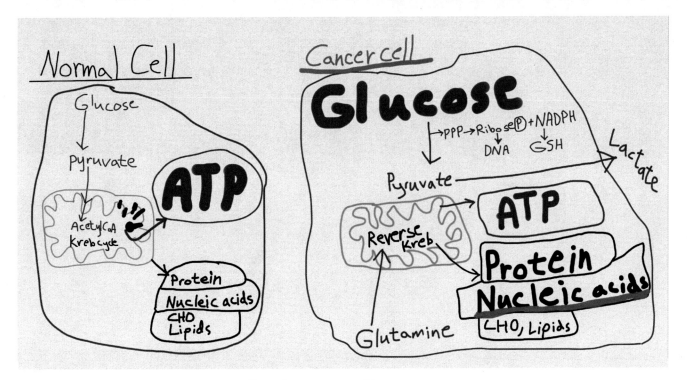

Fig 21: **Comparison of a normal cell and a cancer cell.**
Normal cell = worker = priority is make ATP → so can do more work

Cancer cell = grower = priority is biosynthesis → must double itself to replicate

Normal cell has a job to do. Eg. a liver cell needs to make bile, to de-toxify chemicals, to excrete estrogenic chemicals, to maintain a normal blood glucose level during fasting.

Liver is the metabolic workhorse of the human body. Liver cells need to make lots of ATP (Adenosine TriPhosphate) to provide energy for all that work. ATP is like the "twenty dollar bill" energy currency for getting things done inside a cell.

Cancer cells have damaged mitochondria. Mitochondria need oxygen for making ATP. Lack of oxygen is called hypoxia. Hypoxia damages mitochondria. Damaged mitochondria cannot make much ATP.

Hypoxia kills most cells. With hypoxia, sometimes a cell survives by transforming its metabolism from aerobic (oxygen using) to anaerobic (functioning without oxygen).

Cancer cells do NOT want to do any useful work. Cancer cells are like the Johhny Paycheck song, they just say, "Take this job & shove it. I ain't working for you no more."

Cancer cells are like an anaerobic bacteria. Cancer cell only want one thing = replication.

Before it can replicate, a cancer cell needs to "double itself" = to make copies of all its protein, DNA, RNA & membrane lipids.

A human cell has 3.3 billion base pairs of DNA. It takes a lot of carbon building blocks to make 3.3 billion nucleic acids (the building blocks for making DNA.

In order to replicate itself, a cancer cell needs lots of the amino acids, leucine and methionine; a cancer cell needs lots of iron; a cancer cell needs lots of lipids (fats).

Question: What would I do?

Answer: **Deprive the cancer of leucine, methionine, iron & lipids!!**

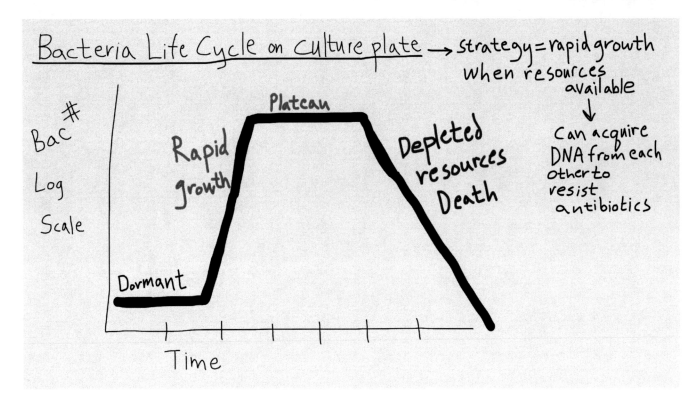

Fig 22: **Bacteria life cycle** = just wants to grow as fast as possible. Bacteria replicates as fast as it can, then uses up its resources, and dies. Rather stupid. Cancer tries to do the same thing = grow as rapidly as possible, and then kill the patient. Luckily, there are many things that might slow down the growth of cancer.

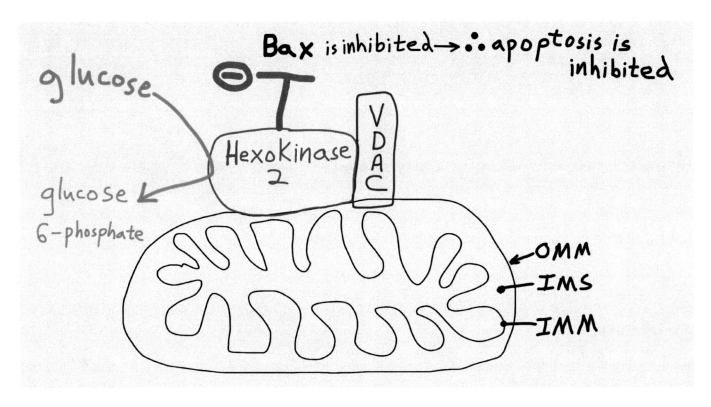

Fig 23: **The key metabolic change in a cancer cell is upregulation (increase) in Hexokinase 2 (HK2).** HK2 stabilizes the outer mitochondrial membrane (OMM), and blocks BAX. This prevents apoptosis; ie. this prevents the cancer cell from dying. This helps to make the cancer cell to become relatively immortal.

The pattern of changes in a cancer cell are focused on rapid, anaerobic growth, and then spreading to other locations. This might be an old school trick from primitive cells, around from the early days of the earth, when the atmospheric oxygen supply might have been intermittent. Ie. having a backup set of enzymes that enable the cell to make energy during low oxygen conditions.

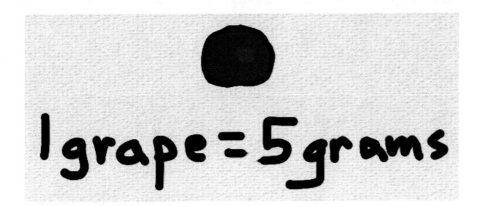

Fig 24: One grape is 5 grams.

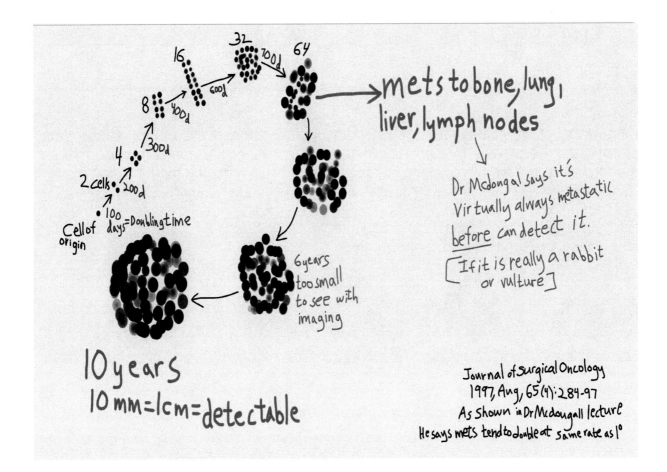

Fig 25: Even small **cancers tend to shed a lot of cells into the blood.**

A 1 gram tumor can shed **over a million cancer cells into the blood in one day.**

Immune system is needed to remove cancer cells.

Therefore you want to PROTECT your immune system!

Ref: Quantitation of cell shedding into efferent blood of mammary adenocarcinoma" Thomas Butler, Cancer Res, March 1, 1975, 35, 3, 512-6

Chemo tends to suppress the immune system.

How is the body going to control the tumor if the immune system is suppressed?

This a major problem with chemo.

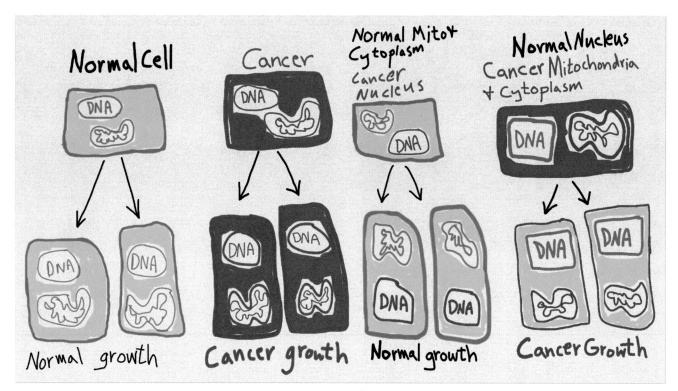

Fig 26: **Thomas Seyfried Phd did a brilliant experiment to show that cancer "comes from" the mitochondria & cytoplasm** (consistent with the metabolic theory of cancer); and not from the nuclear DNA (which is what one would suspect if the somatic mutation theory of cancer were correct). Thomas Seyfried Phd, book "Cancer as a metabolic disease," c. 2012.

The first cell, all in green, is a normal cell; when it replicates it makes 2 normal copies of itself. Second cell is a cancer cell that also can replicate.

Third column is a "hybrid" cell with the mitochondria and cytoplasm from a normal cell, but with the DNA from a cancer cell. This cell replicates NORMALLy!! Hybrid cells are called Cybrids = Cell + h-ybrid

The last column is a cell with normal nuclear DNA, but with mitochondria and cytoplasm from a cancer cell.

The cell with normal nuclear DNA, but abnormal mitochondria and cytoplasm replicates as a cancer!!!

Ie. the cancer causing part of the cell was the cytoplasm and mitochondria & NOT the nuclear DNA.

This is what the metabolic theory of cancer (MTC) predicts. This is another reason why the MTC is useful.

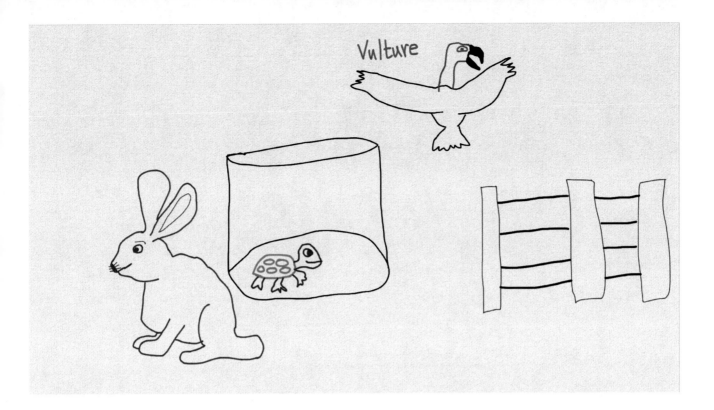

Fig 27: **The three categories of cancer** according to George Crile MD & Gilbert Welch MD.

Rabbit = what people think of when they hear the word "cancer."

Vultures = very rare, highly aggressive cancers, that kill the patient quickly.

Most cancers are turtles → get "over detected" with screening = major pitfall of screening.

Imagine that you own a farm that is 100 square miles big. In the center, there is fenced in enclosure" with rabbits, turtles and vultures, that represent different types of cancer.

If the vulture gets out of the enclosure, it will fly off the farm so fast, that you won't know what happened. **Vultures are VERY rare.** You can't screen for a vulture, because it will pop up, and kill the patient, between screening intervals.

Everyone" thinks cancer is a **rabbit**. That you MUST stop it from running to the fence. Rabbits are the cancers that get treated most often with chemo and surgery.

A **turtle** is a tumor that grows so slowly, that it won't kill the patient. For many turtles it's best to just follow them up with zero invasive treatment

Here's the big secret. Most cancers are turtles!

You DON'T want to treat a turtle with chemo. For turtles, the chemo is worse than the tumor.

Lots of prostate "carcinomas" are turtles. You don't want to surgerize a turtle, unless you've got a good reason.

Prostatectomy (surgical removal of prostate) can cause impotence and urinary incontinence and pain.

You don't want to risk your Johnson & your tinkle for a turtle!

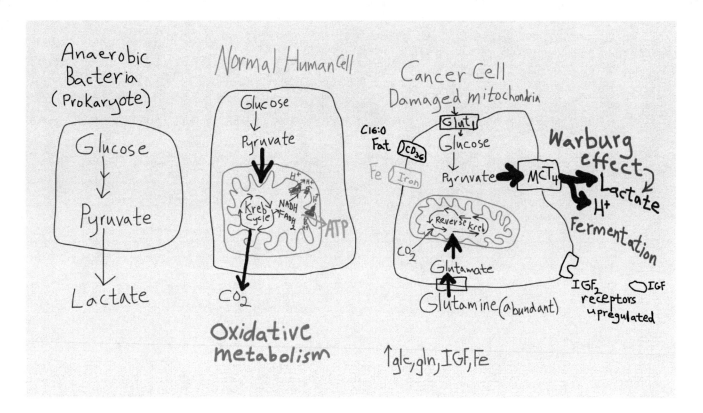

Fig 28: **Cancer metabolism and the tumor milieu** = microenvironment.

This is one of the most important pages in the book. Feel free to fold over the page corner, or to put a post it on it. You're gonna wanna come back to this page.

Cancer is not a single mutation; it's a **WHOLE NEW TYPE OF LIFE.**

Cancer cell upregulates (increases) glucose (glut1) transporters. Cancer cells can burn t hrough 100x more glucose than normal cells. That's why PET scans are positive; because the cancer takes up lots of glucose.

Cancer cells upregulate glutamine receptors. Glutamine is the most common amino acid. The cancer cells can often run almost all of their metabolism form glutamine. That's a major reason why, in my opinion, keto type diets are unlikely to be helpful for cancer patients.

Cancer cells upregulate iron receptors (called "Transferrin" receptors), because cancer cells need lots of iron for replication.

Cancer cell upregulate receptors for Insulin Like Growth Factor (IGF or ILGF). Things that increase IGF, like high fat diets, tend to increase the risk of cancer growth.

Cancer cell pumps protons into the extracellular space = the space just outside the cell. This acidifies the extracellular space.

Acidification of the extracellular space helps to suppress the immune system. It also helps the cancer cell to outcompete the neighboring, normal cells, which are more dependent on oxygen.

Lessons learned:

1. I would avoid the chronic hyperglycemia of diabetes, which is mostly caused by excess dietary fat.

2. I would avoid excess dietary protein, especially animal protein.

3. I would avoid excess dietary iron. I would even donate blood, to keep my serum ferritin somewhere like 25-70.

4. I would avoid things that tend to acidify the blood, like animal protein and sodium chloride (salt), because the chloride tends to displace bicarbonate (a pH buffer) out of the blood.

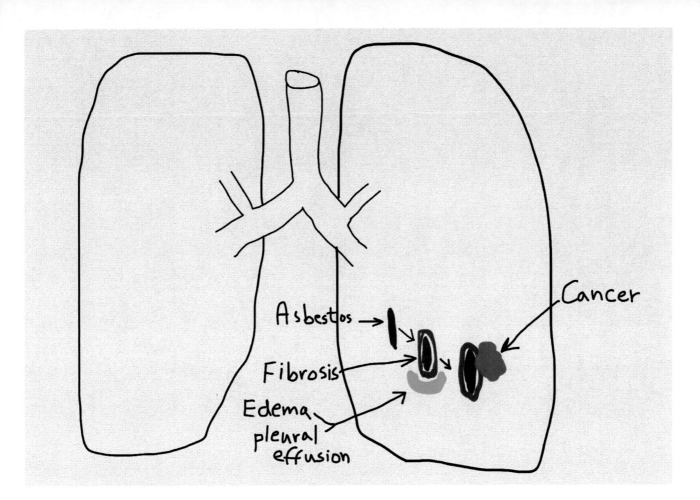

Fig 29: **Warburg effect = MTC** (Metabolic Theory of Cancer) → tissue hypoxia causes cancer. Person inhales a fiber of asbestos. The asbestos is recognized as foreign by the immune system; this causes inflammation. The inflammation walls off the asbestos fiber. Some normal cells get "stuck" in the inflammatory debris.

Scar tissue = mostly collagen (also in this context called "fibrosis"). A bulky scar forms around the asbestos fiber. Some normal lung cells get trapped in the scar.

The scar partially blocks oxygen delivery. This drop in oxygen, because of the scarring around the asbestos fiber, can cause anaerobic transformation of the enveloped cells, eg. into a cancer called mesothelioma

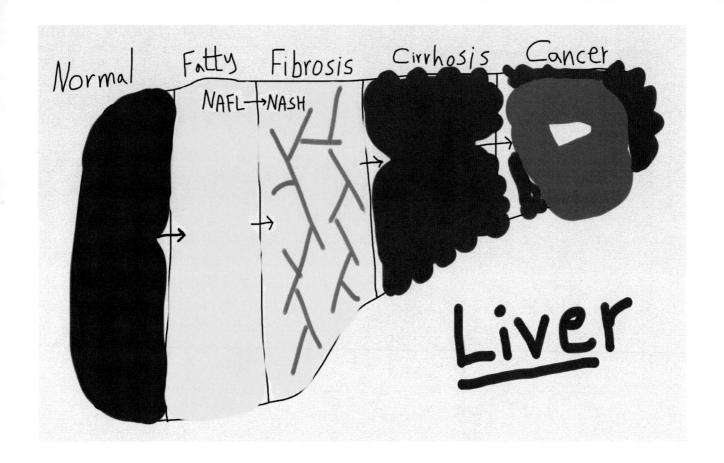

Fig 30: **Warburg effect** = **MTC** (Metabolic Theory of Cancer) → tissue hypoxia causes cancer.

Same mechanism here. Scarring in the liver due to fatty liver – or to alcohol – or to hepatitis virus: generates production of collagen (fibrosis).

The fibrosis blocks oxygen delivery to normal cells. Most of these cells will die, but some will transform into functioning like anaerobic bacteria = will become cancer.

The name "Warburg" comes from Otto Warburg Phd, a German biochemist, who won the Nobel Prize in 1931. He discovered the **"Warburg effect."**

The Warburg effect is the finding that when cells are deprived of oxygen, they don't all die. Some are transformed into anaerobic metabolism = some become cancer.

Warburg's research was largely forgotten during the 2nd half of the 1900's. All the big money in cancer research was based on the SMT (Somatic Mutation Theory) of cancer.

The problem with the SMT is that the data does not support it. Nowadays, it's relatively easy to determine the sequence of DNA, and to map out a pattern of mutations.

The SMT suggests that a cancer cell will go through a characteristic, predictable pattern of mutations on its path of transformation from normal into cancer.

This was tested in the The Cancer Genome Atlas (TCGA = the bases of DNA) project. The SMT failed.

The mutation patterns were relatively random (as predicted by the MTC = Metabolic Theory of Cancer). This indicates that the mutations happened later, sort of largely after the cell had become cancerous.

The MTC also explains the risk factors for cancer better than the SMT. Eg. In 1970's the Papua New Guinea and Japanese smoked tobacco about as much as Americans, but had much less cancer. Why?

Because the Americans were eating a high fat diet with lots of animal protein! Unlike the Papuans who were eating mostly sweet potatos (only 4.5% fat) or the Japanese, eating mostly rice (only 1% fat).

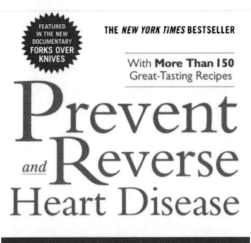

Fig 31: **Dr Esselstyn's book "Prevent & reverse heart disease"** is a masterpiece. 198 patients in a row, who FOLLOWED the diet, had ZERO cardiovascular events.

It doesn't get any better than that! Everything else, including coronary artery stents, coronary artery bypass graft (CABG) surgery, DASH diet, Mediterranean diet are a joke compared to Esselstyn diet for treatment of chronic, coronary artery atherosclerosis.

The Esselstyn diet = 100% vegan = no meat (not one bite!); no dairy (not one drop!); no oil (not one drop! & that includes no olive oil!), no sweets, no caffeine.

Why is Esselstyn's diet mentioned in this book about preventing cancer? **Because, Esselstyn's diet improves blood flow; improved blood flow means better tissue oxygenation;** better tissue oxygenation means better chance to prevent the Warburg effect of cancer causation; and better chance to prevent the hypoxic milieu that is associated with cancer growth.

"Coronary artery disease is virtually nonexistent in Tarahumara, Papua New Guinea, Okinawa, Central Africa, and rural China.

Nitric oxide is the most powerful vasodilator in the body.

Nitric oxide is the life jacket of your arteries.

The number one goal of good arterial function is to maintain adequate amounts of nitric oxide.

As we get older, our arteries produce less nitric oxide.

But the body has another way to produce nitric oxide: from plants.

Eat green vegetables at every meal to keep your arteries bathed in nitric oxide."

- Dr Caldwell Esselstyn.

Sunshine also increases systemic, arterial, nitric oxide!

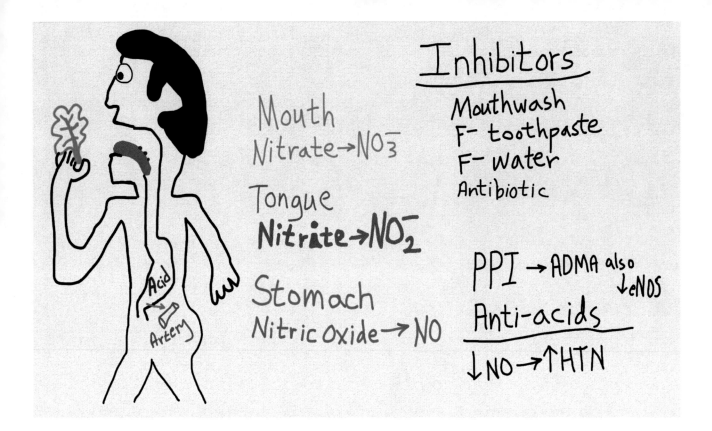

Fig 32: **Conversion of dietary plant nitrates (NO₂⁻) to systemic nitric oxide (NO).**

Green vegetables like salad contain nitrates, NO_3^-.

Bacteria on tongue convert the nitrates to nitrite, NO_2^-.

In the stomach, the stomach acid converts the nitrite to nitric oxide, NO.

Nitric oxide is absorbed into the blood, and has a systemic vasodilator effect; ie. it dilates arteries.

Dilated arteries provide more blood flow, at a lower blood pressure.

Ie. eating leafy greens helps to dilate arteries; optimize blood pressure; prevent atherosclerosis; improve tissue oxygenation; lower the risk of hypoxia related, Warburg effect, cancer causation.

Ie. lower the risk of a tumor related, hypoxic milieu. Milieu = microenvironment.

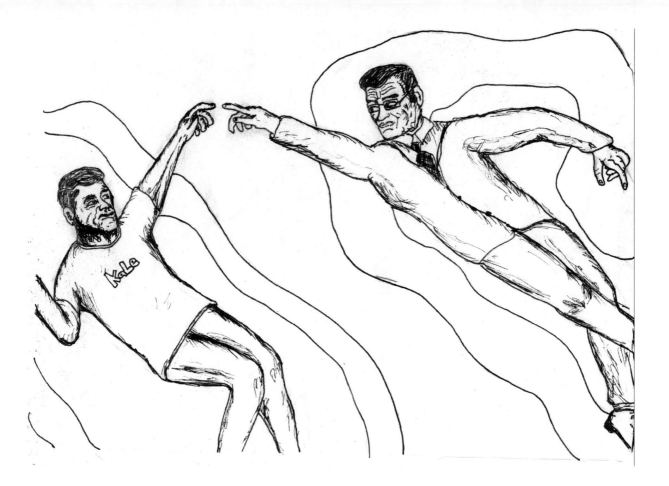

Fig 33: **Dr Esselstyn portrayed like the Old Testament God** in Michelangelo's painting of "Creation of Adam" on the ceiling of the Sistine Chapel in the Vatican in Rome. The OT God is not like Jesu Christu who forgives you for most of your mischief & idiocy.

The OT God says, "Obey my commandments, or I will kick your ass!"

Dr Esselstyn says, "Follow the diet, or your arteries will get plugged up, and that is like an ass kicking."

By the way, the Dr Kempner rice diet, the Dr Mcdougall diet, the Chef AJ WF PBD with no SOFA's, Ruth Heidrich Phd diet, Lorraine Day vegan diet, Janet Murray-Wakelin raw vegan diet, Dr Rogers "Spartan Vegan" diet are all very similar.

They are all: Low fat, 100% vegan. That includes no dairy. No oil.

Kempner's diet was the most limited in food choice = Rice as the only starch.

Ruth Heidrich, Janet Murray-Wakelin, Lorraine Day tend to eat a lot of fruits, and thus a lot of "raw" = uncooked food. There are some who believe that raw food is healthier.

Dr Mcdougall believes that starch is the best food for humans, and that they should get the vast majority of their calories from starch. Dr Mcdougall recommends limiting fruits to about 1-3 servings per day.

Esselstyn, Mcdougall, AJ allow non-organic food.

Rogers diet is only organic food, with no MSG, MfG, aspartame, and no cooking on aluminum, iron or POFA cookware. And no iron enriched foods. Rogers eats about 60% starch, 35% fruits, 5% veggies (in terms of calories).

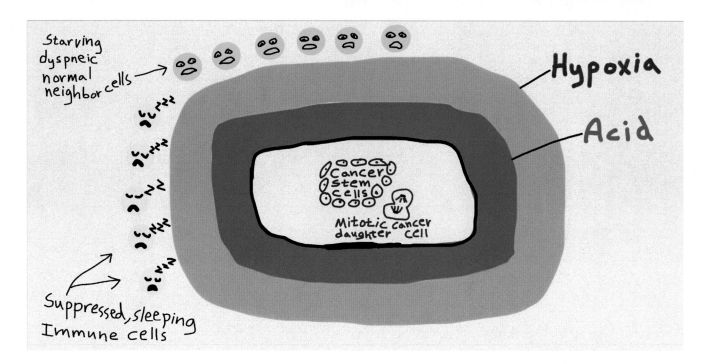

Fig 34: <u>**Tumor milieu**</u> **= hypoxic & acidotic!** The yellow "faces" are suppressed immune cells that are "put to sleep" by the peri-tumoral acidity = acidity of the tumor milieu = tumor microenvironment.

The green "faces" are the normal, adjacent cells which are starving due to the peritumoral hypoxia, and because the tumor sucks up most to the local glucose and iron.

Cancer Stem Cells (CSC's) are < 1% of cells in a tumor.

A tumor is more like a colony of cells, than a clone of cells.

Old research often in 2D, monoculture of "cancer" cells.

Modern research, more often, with more realistic, 3D models of tumors.

CSC's are often RESISTANT to chemotherapy!

CSC might initially be replicating slowly, might have more plasma membrane transporters to pump out the drug

Fruits & vegetables are relatively alkaline = favors normal cells, & helps immune system

Meat & Na+Cl- are acidic = favors cancer & suppresses immune system.

Meat is acidic because has an excess of sulfur containing amino acids like methionine and cysteine.

NaCl is acidic, because the chloride accumulates in the blood. The body must maintain a fixed ratio of blood anions (negatively charged ions) relative to cations (positively charged ions).

So, when a person eats lots of salt, the excess chloride (it's an anion), displaces bicarbonate (it's also an anion) from the blood.

Bicarbonate is a pH buffer. When bicarbonate levels are reduced, the blood becomes more acidic. Ie. excess dietary salt (as in sodium chloride) causes a low grade acidosis.

The concern is that this low grade acidosis – by the way, low grade means "mild" – is thought to favor maintained acidity of the tumor microenvironment.

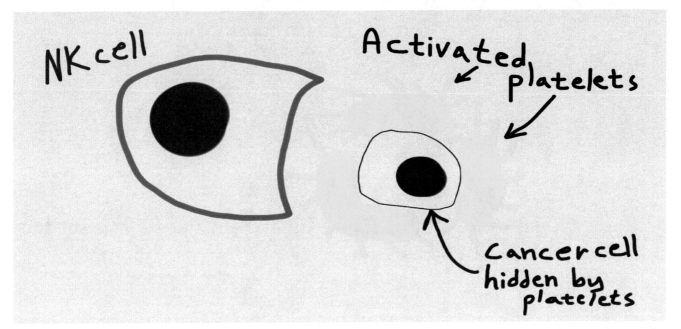

Fig 35: **Stress activates platelets** → activated platelets are more "sticky." Sticky platelets tend to stick to things like cancer cells in the blood. **Activated platelets can hide cancer cells from the immune system.**

When platelets stick to cancer cells, they cover up the outer surface of the cancer cell. This is a problem, because the cancer cells are then "HIDDEN" from the immune system.

Immune cells are like an ID card checkpoint.

The immune cells rub against the surface of other cells in the blood, and "check" their outer surface "sugar-acid-proteins."

The more medically precise way to say "sugar-acid-proteins" is to call them sialic acid residues on the proteo-glycans of the cancer cell's outer surface, glyco-calyx.

Glyco means sugar. Calyx means coating. Proteo means protein.

Sialic acids can be thought of as sugars with an acid group attached. Sorry for all the verbiage, but the terminology is here so that if you ever want to look it up, it's readily available.

The key point is that excessive stress is bad, because it makes platelets sticky, and then they can potentially hide cancer cells from the immune system.

Stress equivalents are things that have the same effect as stress = elevate the same hormones as stress = elevate cortisol and catecholamines.

Cortisol is the cortico-steroid hormone that raises blood glucose levels during stress. Cortisol also suppresses the immune system.

Catecholamines are adrenaline (aka epinephrine) and noradrenaline (aka norepinephrine). Catecholamines are of concern, because they can potentially function as sidero-phores.

Sidero = iron. Phore = to transfer. Sidero-phore = a molecule that transports iron.

Ie. catecholamines are thought to potentially function as sidero-phores, increasing the risk of iron molecules being delivered to cancer cells (and to bacterial cells).

Stress equivalents include lack of sleep and caffeine and corticosteroid medications, because all of these cause increased blood cortisol and catecholamines.

High dietary sodium and high saturated fat can also cause activation of platelets.

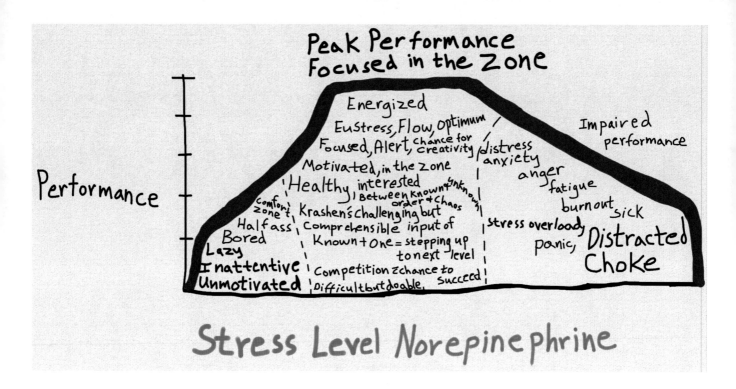

Fig 36: **Yerkes Dodson curve of stress vs performance.** Too little stress and you're bored, lazy, half assed, not interested, unmotivated.

Too much stress is stress overload, or distress; you're distracted, anxious, and eventually fatigued, or even burnt out.

Optimal stress is when you're in the zone. The task is challenging, but doable. Your working on the edge between the known and the unknown.

The peak performance stress level is where you want to be when you are exercising or doing some other interesting task.

For mundane things, like doing the laundry, and so on, you don't need any stress, because these tasks are so easy to do.

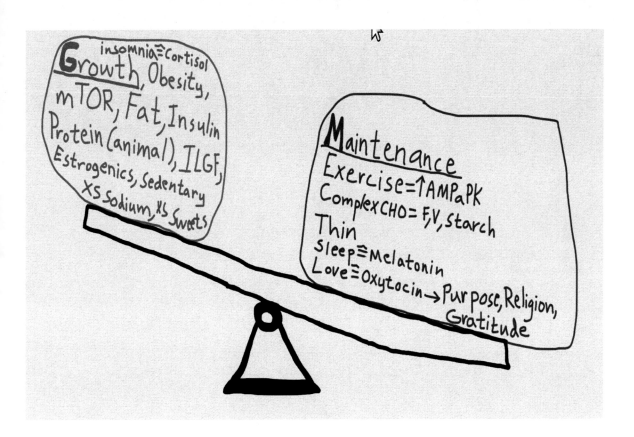

Fig 37: Cell phases of growth vs maintenance. You want to spend as much time in MAINTENANCE as possible.

If you are a 20 year old body builder, then animal protein, with its extra leucine and methionine can increase mTOR activation to increase your rate of cell growth and replication.

If you are over 30, or have cancer then you do NOT want to activate mTOR.

MTOR is a nutrient sensing pathway that is like a **building contractor.** Building contractor needs to make sure all the building materials are available, before it can build.

Rate limiting steps most commonly are leucine and methionine, but can also be a lack of available iron or lipids. Good! You want their to be relatively little available leucine, methionine, iron & lipid.

You want to slow down mTOR!

Activation of mTOR also accelerates aging, because it speeds up arrival at the Hayflick limit.

Hayflick was a molecular biologist who worked with tissue cultures. He found that human somatic cells - cells of the body that were not stem cells or germ cells – would only divide about 60 times, and then die.

The apparent reason for these cells dying is because they lack the telomerase enzyme. Telomerase is used to maintain the ends of chromosomes. Without telomerase enzyme, the chromosome of a somatic cell will shorten with each cell division. It shortens, because of the mechanism of DNA replication in somatic cells.

By exercising, you shut off mTOR, and turn on the AMPK (Adenosine Monophosphate Protein Kinase) pathway. That's good! High ATP levels means high energy for the cell.

High AMP levels means low energy for the cell. When ATP gives off one phosphate, it becomes ADP (Adenosine Di Phosphate). When ATP gives off two phosphates it becomes AMP (Adenosine Mono Phosphate).

AMPK tells the cell, "We are tired. That exercise used up our ATP. We must turn off mTOR, and forget about growing for a while. We need to just focus on restoring our ATP levels."

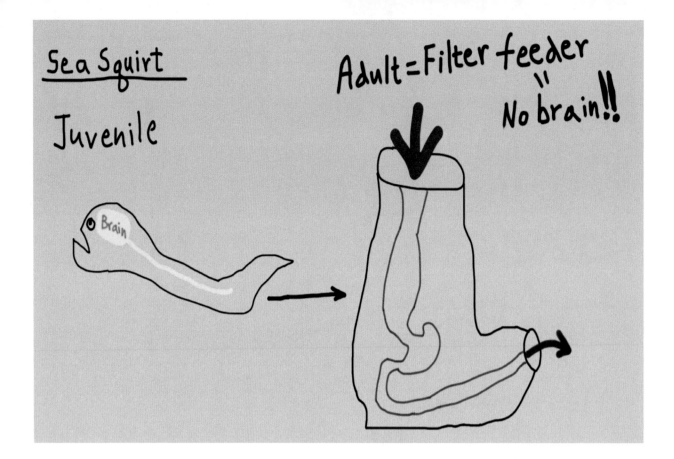

Fig 38: **Exercise improves and maintains cognitive function.**

"Why do animals have brains, but plants do not? Because animals move!" - Voltaire (1694-1778).

What is the purpose of the brain? To be able to walk down a path in a jungle, forest or prairie and survive.

The sea squirt is like a tadpole during its juvenile phase; it has a brain; it swims around.

During adulthood, the sea squirt attaches to a rock, and becomes a filter feeder.

Because it no longer moves around, it does NOT need a brain; it's brain is reabsorbed.

Something similar happens in humans who just sit around watching TV. They become stupider.

Exercise has many benefits for the brain:

Increases BDNF (Brain Derived Neurotrophic growth Factor) = helps neurons to grow & enables formation of new neurons. In the brain, this is a good thing. The brain needs to do this to be able to learn new things.

Increases neurogenesis = formation of new neurons and new synapses. In the brain this is a good thing = needed for learning new things.

Increases brain glycogen storage = a good thing = more energy for the brain.

Increases brain cells mitochondrial biogenesis = a good thing = more energy for the brain.

Improves insulin sensitivity. Exercise causes glucose transporters type 4 to move from cytoplasm up to the plasma membrane. This enables glucose to enter cells.

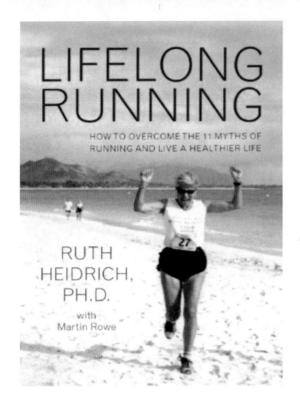

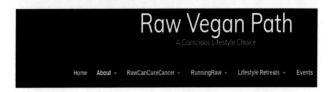

About Us

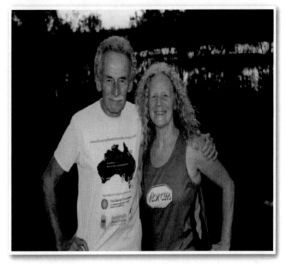

Introducing veteran raw vegan runners Alan Murray and Janette Murray-Wakelin

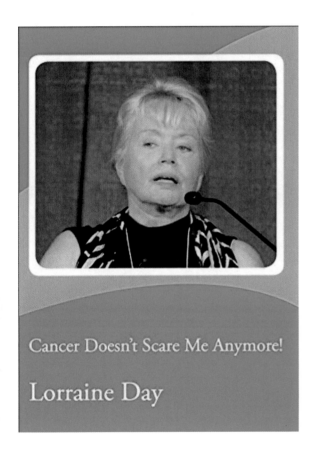

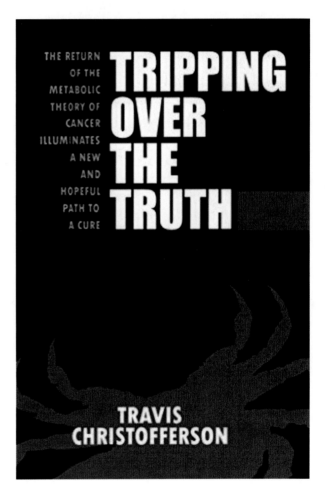

Fig 39: **Great books about preventing and treating cancer.** The book by Janet Murray Wakelin is called "Raw can cure cancer."

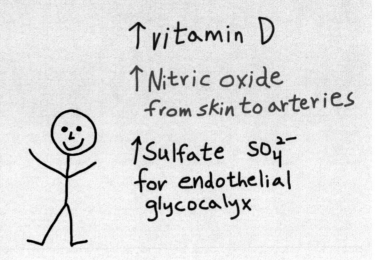

Fig 40: **Sunshine is your friend.**

Sunshine increases vitamin D.

Vitamin D from sunshine is much better than vitamin D from pills.

Sunshine also increases systemic nitric oxide to improve blood flow.

Sunshine also appears to improve sulfation of the endothelial glycocalyx = it helps to keep arteries healthy.

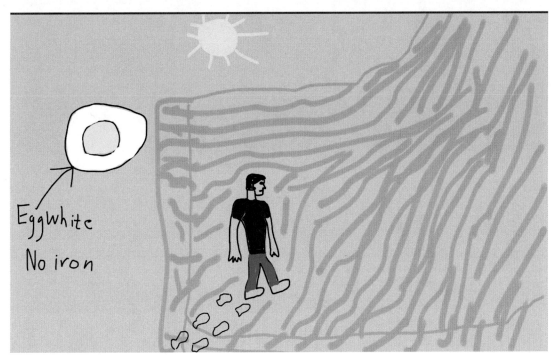

Fig 41: **Cancer needs iron to grow.** Cancer is like an anaerobic bacteria. Bacteria need iron to grow.

With a chicken egg, the eggshell is permeable to air and to bacteria. The chicken embryo is the egg yolk. The egg white is made of protein with almost zero iron.

How come the bacteria can NOT get to the yoke? Because the egg white has almost zero iron!

How come a human cannot go far in the desert? Because there's no water.

By sequestering iron, the human body helps prevent bacteria growth and cancer growth.

By avoiding dietary iron = avoiding meat and iron enriched foods = you help prevent your body from becomining iron overloaded = you help your body to keep iron away from any potential cancer cells.

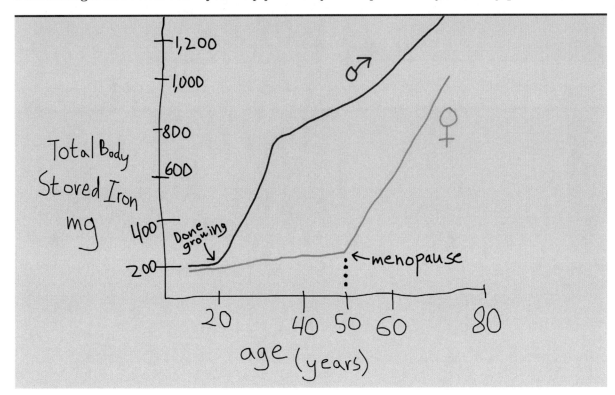

Fig 42: **In Western countries, most men rapidly become iron overloaded after 20 years of age** (ie. after they are done growing physically). Most women, after menopause, rapidly become iron overloaded.

When a person becomes overloaded, they have more free iron. Free iron can cause problems.

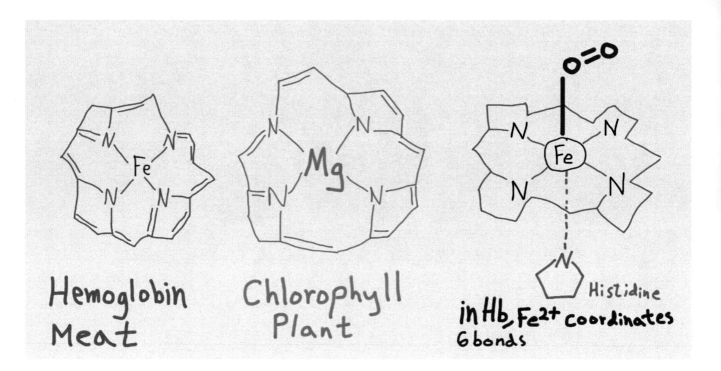

Fig 43: **Iron is located in the center of hemoglobin.** Magnesium is located in the center of chlorophyll.

Meat contains hemoglobin. Hemoglobin contains iron. Meat contains iron.

Magnesium from plants is a good thing. Magnesium is a vasodilator = helps improve blood flow.

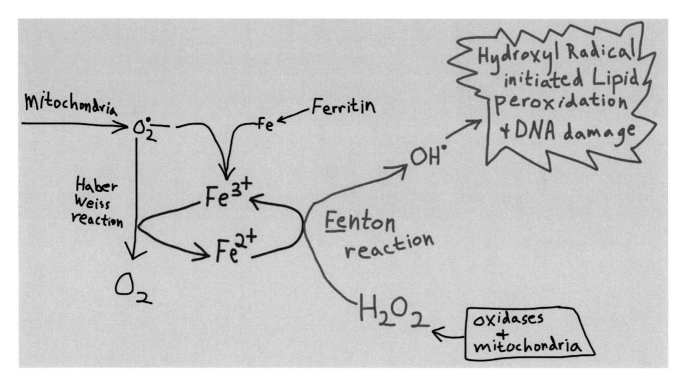

Fig 44: **Ferrous redox cycling** → Fe is NOT a substrate → it's a catalyst → can be autocatalytic → small amount can do damage.

During ferrous redox cycling the iron cycles back and forth between Fe2+ and Fe3+.

As the iron undergoes ferrous redox cycling, it gives off electrons to H2O2, that can be converted into hydroxyl radicals.

The hydroxyl radicals damage tissues including cell membranes and DNA. Damage from hydroxyl radicals increases the risk of cancer.

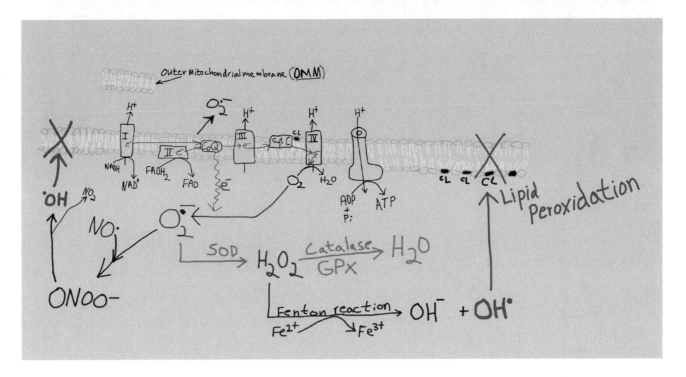

Fig 45: **Mitochondria electron transport chain (ETC).** Drawing shows an electron leaking from the ETC. The electron reacts with oxygen in the mitochondrial matrix to form a superoxide free radical, O2-.

The superoxide is usually quickly neutralized by SOD (Super Oxide Dismutase). However, when there is an excess of electron leak, and there is free iron present in the mitochondrial matrix; then the Fenton reaction can occur.

Ferrous means iron in latin. Fe is the symbol for iron. Fe are the first two letters in Fenton for the Fenton reaction.

The Fenton reaction produces hydroxyl radicals, OH. The hydroxyl radicals can then cause lipid peroxidation damage to the inner mitochondrial membrane (IMM).

Remember that hypoxia damage to mitochondria was the mechanism for the Warburg effect. Well, other causes of mitochondrial injury can also increase the risk of cancer.

<u>**Why is iron overload dangerous**</u>?

Superoxide is normally cleared by SOD & Catalase (or Gpx).

Excess superoxide → **can combine with nitric oxide** → **leading to ONOO-** → **then hydroxyl radical.**

Or can undergo Fenton reaction to also make hydroxyl radical → then can cause **lipid peroxidation.**

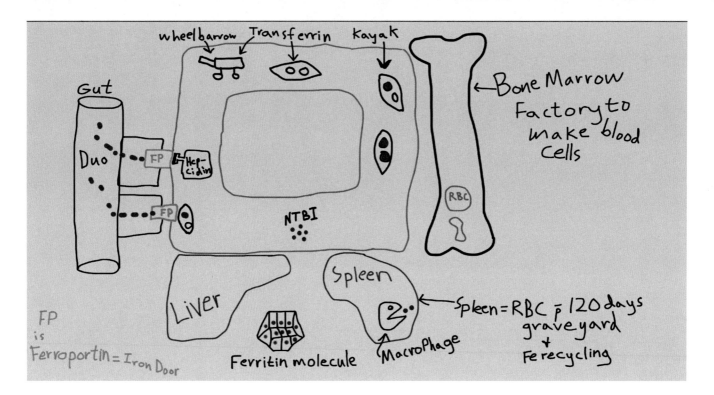

Fig 46: **Iron metabolism.** Iron is absorbed from the duodenum, into the duodenal enterocyte. Gut is called the enteric tract; so gut lining cells are called enterocytes.

Duodenal enterocytes can store iron for a few days. When the body wants the iron, an iron transport protein in the blood called Transferrin, will bind to the inner side (AB-luminal) of the duodenocyte.

The iron will exit the duodenocyte by passing through FerroPortin. FerroPortin means iron door. Transferrin will then carry the iron to it's destination.

Human cells, especially liver cells, have an iron storage protein called Ferritin. One molecule of Ferritin can bind to 4,500 molecules of iron.

So the human body can store a lot of iron. The body stores iron so that in case the person has bleeding, the red blood cells can have their hemoglobin rapidly replenished.

Iron was relatively scarce to our ancestors. Iron is overly abundant to modern people.

Westerners have a tendency to be iron overloaded; and this increases the risk of oxidative stress and cancer.

Smart move is to reduce iron levels = serum ferritin levels to about 25-80 by #1. NEVER eat meat. #2. avoid other high iron foods like iron "enriched" grains & cereals. #3. if have well water, then remove iron with an iron filter. #4. Do not use iron cookware.

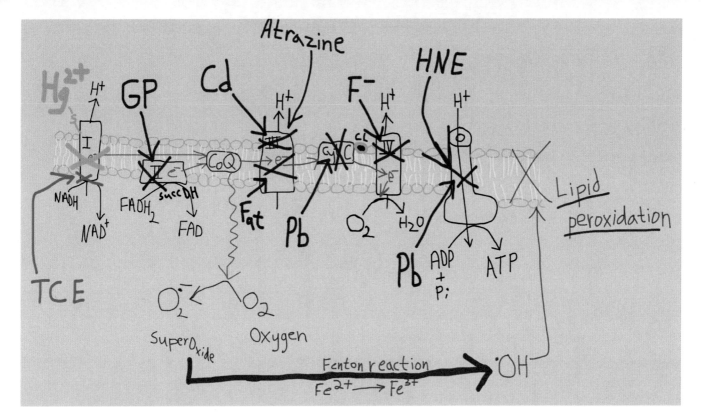

Fig: 47: **Mitochondrial toxins:** Avoid all these as best you can. I made separate videos about all of these available at you tube channel "Peter Rogers MD." If you tube ever gives me the boot, I will put all of these videos on Rumble, Bitchute & other sites.

- Hg = mercury
- TCE = TriChloroEthylene = dry cleaning, etc
- GP = Gly-phosphate = nonorganic foods like soy, etc
- Cd = Cadmium
- Atrazine
- Fat
- Pb = lead,
- F- = fluoride
- HNE = Hydroxynonenal
- Excess iron
- Insulin resistance in the brain (a/w MAM's = Mitochondrial Associated Membranes of the endoplasmic reticulum)

Why is it so hard to learn nutrition?

It's easy to learn what to eat = starches, fruits, veggies

The hard part is un-learning all the incorrect stuff you've heard all your life

Here's the good stuff that you should eat:

Starches = rice, potatos, sweet potatos, oatmeal, quinoa, beans, wheat

Fruits = blueberries, watermelon, bananas, papaya, etc.

Vegetables = salads, cauliflower, kale, etc.

100% organic.

Whole foods with the exception of oatmeal or quinoa.

Only drink filtered water.

No caffeine, no alcohol, no MSG, no oil, no sweets, no added Fe.

Only supplement I take is Vitamin B12 in the form of methyl cobalamin.

Many have given up on learning nutrition, because so much contradictory information on internet.

Many are reluctant to accept that previously they were wrong

Social thinking is good for social, but not for health or achievement. Eg moderation in health is for chumps. Smart person does not just "cut down on meat," they NEVER eat it.

Many don't want to admit that they are fat & unhealthy → often cognitively slow.

Many are shocked that **most so called "experts" are phonies & that Dr's do not know nutrition.**

All university medical centers that I've seen recommend some variation of Mediterranean diet
the **illusion of dietary treatment** = the **Anti-Christ of nutrition,** because it
promises to save people, but doesn't deliver.

After Mediterranean diet fails → patient feels they have no other options →

& they "submit" to lifelong drugs → & eventual surgery.

The system **"milks"** them for money → every day for the rest of their lives.

They end up fat, sick & broke → until they die.

Don't let that happen to you!

The health care system does not like low fat, low sodium vegans, because no one makes money off them.

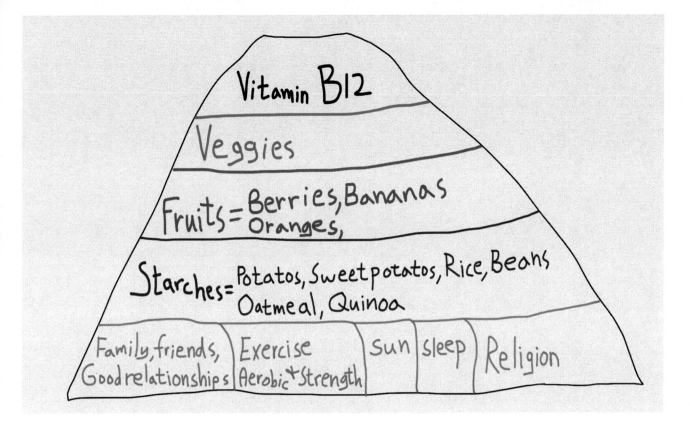

Fig 48: **Spartan Vegan = Poor Man's pyramid of health.**

These are the best foods to eat.

Healthiest populations have close communities of families, friends, religious members.

They exercise every day doing things like walking, growing food, preparing food, taking care of the children.

They get sunshine.

They get adequate sleep, eg. 7-8 hours per night.

They pray or somehow participate in their religion.

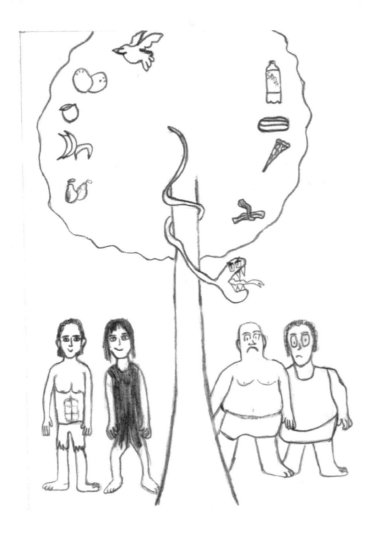

Fig 49: **Choose foods from tree of life= right side.   Avoid foods from tree of death = left side.**

"In the beginning, God created the Heaven and the earth." - Genesis 1:1.

"And God said, let there be light, and there was light." - Genesis 1:3.

"And God saw the light and that it was good; and God divided the light from the darkness." - Genesis 1:4.

"And the Lord God planted a garden eastward in Eden; and there he put the man whom he had formed." - Genesis 1:8.

"So God created man in His own image; in the image of God He created he him; male and female, created he them." - Genesis 1:27.

Before the flood, (Genesis 9:3), men & animals did not eat any animal food, or any processed food.

 "Then God said, "Behold, I have given you every plant yielding seed, which is upon the face of all the earth, and every tree which has fruit; it shall be food for you. And to every beast of the earth, and every bird of the air and every creature that crawls upon the earth, I have given every green plant for food." - Genesis 1:29-30.

"And God said, "If thou will hearken to the voice of the Lord thy God, and … wilt give ear to his commandments… I will put none of these diseases upon thee, which I brought upon the Egyptians [low carb Paleos]: for I am the Lord God who heals you." - Exodus 15:26.

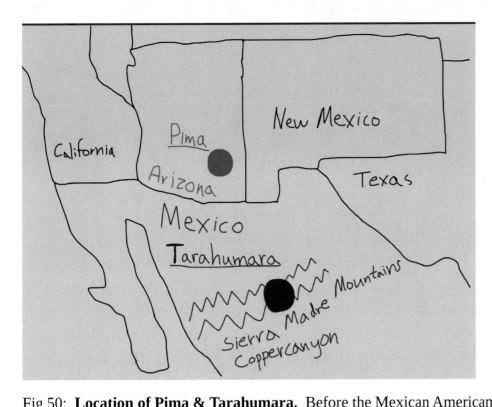

Fig 50: **Location of Pima & Tarahumara.** Before the Mexican American war in 1848, the Pima & Tarahumara were related populations, demographically similar.

Then Pima were absorbed into Arizona, and they now eat the SAD (Standard American Diet) diet.

Tarahumara have largely kept to their traditional diet of corn, beans, squash & local greens.

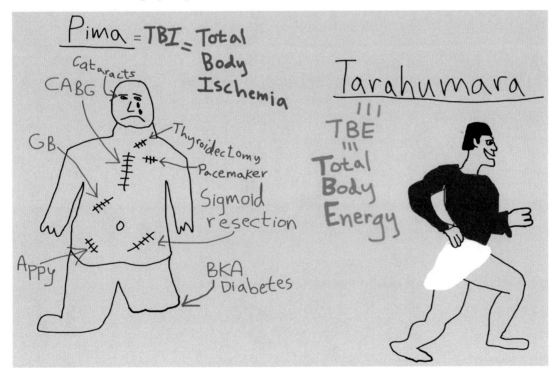

Fig 51: **Pima have lots of obesity & all the other Western diseases** like hypertension, atherosclerosis, impotence, coronary artery disease, gallstones, peripheral vascular disease (treated by amputations), appendicitis, diverticulitis, etc. CABG is Coronary Artery Bypass Graft.

Tarahumara are famous for being ultramarathon runners. They have super endurance, and can run 100 miles in two days. They eat a **low fat plant diet.** Nutrition genius, Nathan Pritikin was so impressed by the Tarahumara, that he patterned his diet after them.

Pritikin wrote "There's no natural diet that's too low in fat… fat is bad."

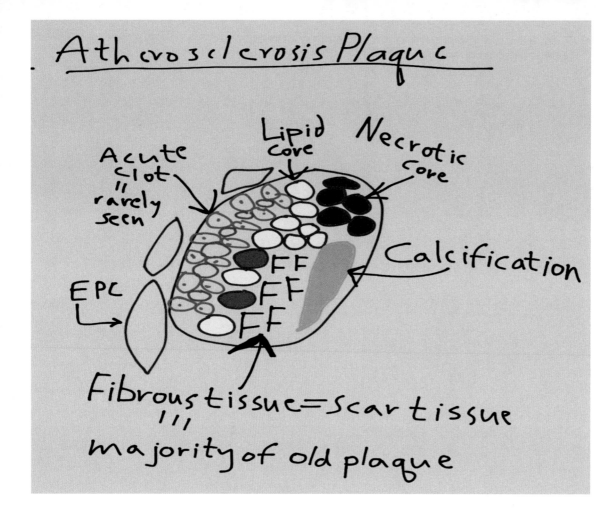

Fig 52: **Atherosclerosis plaque.** Atherosclerosis is partially reversible. The lipid core, necrotic core, early thrombus (= blood clot) component can all be re-absorbed.

The cellular part of the fibrous tissue can be partially reabsorbed.

The acellular part of the fibrous tissue = scar tissue = lots of collagen, cannot be reabsorbed. The calcifications cannot be reabsorbed.

Ability to reabsorb part of the atherosclerotic plaque is a big deal, because a small increase in diameter, leads to a big increase in blood flow: because amount of blood flow is proportional to radius to the fourth power = r^4.

I have lectures about atherosclerosis at you tube channels Peter Rogers MD & at Chef AJ. Chef AJ is the most famous vegan you tube channel.

The atherosclerosis lecture by William Roberts MD on atherosclerosis is also good.

In addition, when a person eats low fat, low sodium vegan, they make life better for the arterial lining cells, called the endothelium.

The endothelium makes the vasodilator called "Nitric Oxide," that's usually labeled "NO."

Vasodilation means to dilate the artery. A dilated artery provides more blood flow.

Better blood flow delivers more oxygen to the tissues, and helps to prevent cancer.

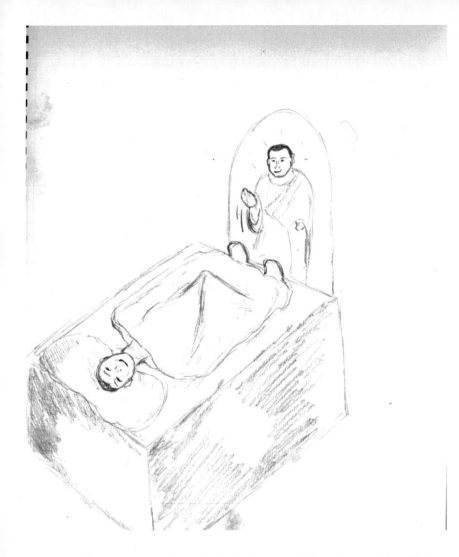

Fig 53: **The resurrection of the Johnson of Lazarus.** Not all, but many male patients have improved potency upon changing to a low fat, low sodium, whole food, vegan diet.

"Jesus came to the tomb of Lazarus. It was a cave with a stone laid across the entrance.

"Take away the stone," Jesus said.

"Lord, by now he stinks" said Martha, the sister of the dead man. "It has already been four days."

Jesus replied, "Did I not tell you that if you believed you would see the glory of God?"

So they took away the stone. Then Jesus lifed his eyes upward and said, "Father, I thank You that You have heard Me. I know that you always hear Me, but I say this for the benefit of the people standing here, so they may believe that You sent Me."

After Jesus said this, He called out in a loud voice, "Lazarus, come out!"

The man who had been dead came out with his hands and feet bound in strips of linen, and his face wrapped in a cloth."

"Unwrap him and let him go," Jesus told them. Acts 9:36-43.

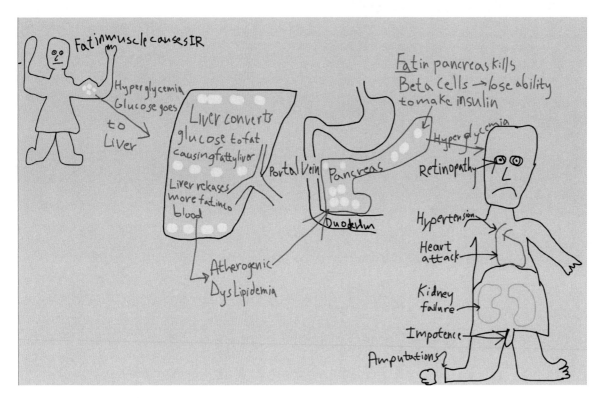

Fig 54: **The stages of diabetes.** Key point is that type 2 diabetes is primarily due to eating excess dietary fat. Dietary fat, especially saturated fat, accumulates in skeletal muscle.

Fat in skeletal muscle causes insulin resistance. Normally, after eating a meal, about 80% of the glucose in the blood goes to the muscle; most of it is stored as glycogen.

The time period that occurs just after eating a meal is called "post prandial." Thus, most postprandial blood glucose goes to skeletal muscle to be stored as glycogen. That's good. That's what you want.

Excess post prandial glucose is also stored in the liver as glycogen.

When fat accumulates in skeletal muscle, it causes "nutrition overload or over nutrition." The fat, saturated fat in particular, causes inhibition of electron transport in mitochondria.

When electron transport is blocked, that is like a traffic jam. The cell senses a problem, and this causes the cell to not want any more glucose to come in.

Normally, glucose type 4 transporters are located in the skeletal muscle cytoplasm, stored in vesicles. When insulin binds to the insulin receptor on the skeletal muscle, plasma membrane; this activates a signal to the glut 4 vesicles, that they should be sent to the plasma membrane.

When glut 4's merge with the plasma membrane, they enable glucose to enter the skeletal muscle cell.

If postprandial glucose can't enter the skeletal muscle, then it accumulates in the blood,causing hyperglycemia (elevated blood glucose).

Hyperglycemia leads to excess glucose in the liver, and eventually to fatty liver. After fatty liver has developed, the pancreas then tends to accumulate too much fat.

When the pancreas becomes fat overloaded, it starts to fail. The beta cells in the pancreas make insulin. As the pancreas accumulates more fat, the beta cells become dysfunctional and/or die. Insulin production drops. The patient becomes an insulin dependent diabetic.

I have videos about diabetes at Peter Rogers MD & Chef AJ you tube channels that go into much more detail.

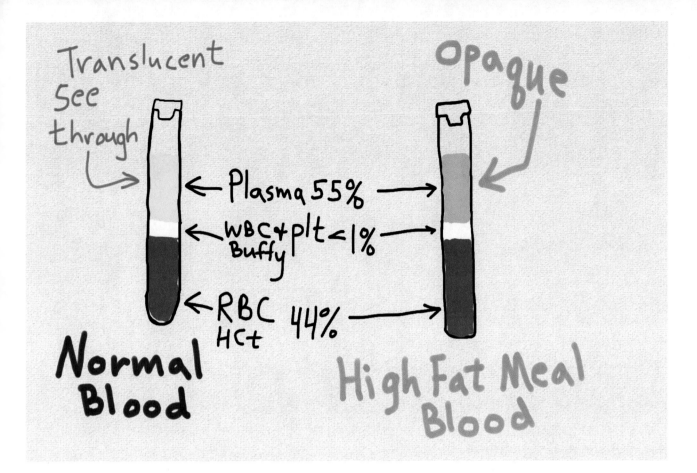

Fig 55: **Dietary fat makes the blood opaque.**

In a test tube, the red blood cells, RBC, layer out on the bottom, and are red.

The white blood cells, WBC, are in the middle, and are called the buffy.

The plasma is on top, and is usually translucent.

The more fat a person eats, the more opaque the plasma becomes.

In general, the more fat a person eats, the more the fat tends to cause the RBC's to stick together in what is called "blood sludge" or rouleaux formation.

Rouleaux means a "stack of coins" in French.

Roueleaux and blood sludge are a way to "thicken" the blood, or to increase blood "viscosity."

Blood sludge-rouleaux is bad, because it decreases oxygen delivery to the tissues.

Things that decrease oxygen delivery to the tissues also increase the risk of cancer.

There is a good scene in the documentary movie called "Game Changers" where they compare test tubes of blood before and after a fatty meal.

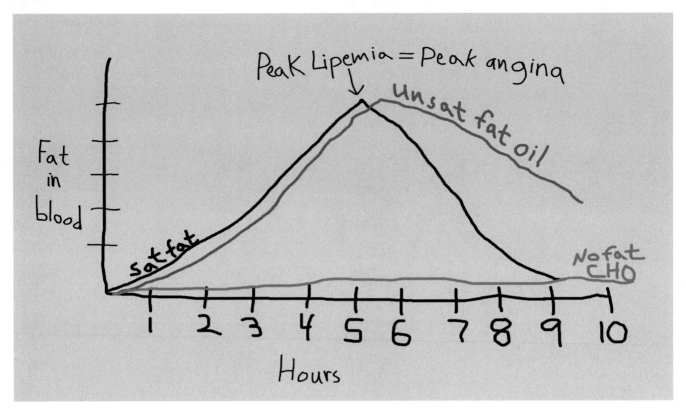

Fig 56: Peter Kuo MD was a cardiologist in Pennsylvania in the 1950's and he **fed his cardiac angina patients a high fat meal with saturated fat.**

Kuo simultaneously measured blood lipids every thirty minutes. At peak lipemia = maximal levels of fat in the blood, the cardiac angina patient would tend to develop chest pain.

Notice how bold, and crazy this experiment is. Nowadays, this experiment would not be allowed. Back in those days, there was no cardiac cath, angioplasty or stenting.

Kuo took patients with known coronary artery atherosclerosis related episodes of chest pain – aka cardiac angina - and fed them a high fat meal; and they tended to develop chest pain at peak lipemia.

In the 1950's Ancel Keys showed that excess dietary saturated fat causes atherosclerosis.

In the 1950's there was a movement to recommend people eat more omega 6 fats – aka polyunsaturated fats (PUFA's) from cooking oils.

Researchers Ran Rosenman and Meyer Friedman showed that eating omega 6 cooking oils caused the same effect as saturated fat had, except that it was worse! More prolonged!

Their research assistants were annoyed, because the experiments began early in the morning, and the patients still had blood sludge into the evening. The research assistants wanted to go home!

The average American dummy who eats 2 or more meals a day with oils is keeping their blood thick all day long = increasing their risk of plugging up their arteries – like in theheart for a heart attack

Dr Kuo also noted that the thick blood causes a 15-20% drop in oxygen delivery to the tissues. Roy Swank noted in hamster brains that a high saturated fat meal caused a 30% drop in oxygen delivery.

Decreased oxygen delivery means increased risk of cancer.

As shown by the green line at the bottom of the graph, the patient who did not eat the high fat meals had zero hyperlipidemia and zero angina.

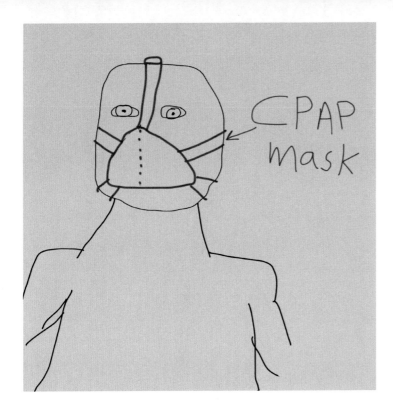

Fig 57: **Obstructive sleep apnea (OSA).** OSA patients are notoriously stupid.

OSA patients are often sleepy during the day.

Theoretically, fat OSA patients have excess fat in their airway that can be partially obstructive when they are sleeping.

Other researchers think that the apnea component of OSA is caused by a neuropathy.

Either way, the OSA patient have relatively poor oxygenation of their blood when sleeping at night.

Researchers put an oxygen sensor on their fingers while the OSA patients are sleeping at night.

The oxygen saturation levels in the blood can drop a lot.

Normally, oxygen saturation levels in the blood are in the mid to high 90's. With sleep apnea patients, I've seen the O2 sat levels drop into the 60's.

How do you think the brain cells respond to a drop in blood oxygen? They don't like it!

Low oxygen is called "hypoxia."

Excess hypoxia means that brain cells cannot get enough oxygen to make energy. If a brain cell cannot get enough oxygen to make energy, it often dies.

Slow death of brain cells due to hypoxia is called "apoptosis." Apoptosis is also called "programmed cell death." Apoptosis means that the cell dies gradually, so that it can recycle itself. Cell recycling means that the cellular components are put into transport vesicles so they can be used by other cells.

In comparison, comple loss of oxygen is called anoxia. Anoxia causes sudden death of a cell. When a big artery in the brain is suddenly occluded, like during a stroke, then brain cells die suddenly, and this is called necrosis.

Lowering dietary fat helps to prevent obesity, diabetes and OSA. This is another way that a low fat diet helps to improve oxygen delivery to tissues, and help prevent cancer.

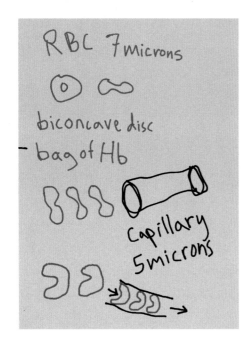 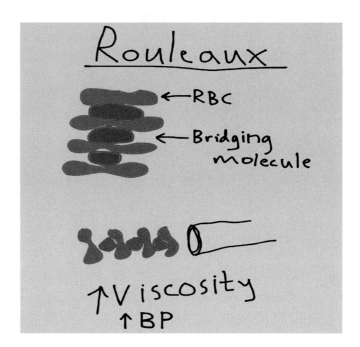

Figures 58 & 59: **Typical RBC is about 7 microns. Typical capillary is about 5 microns.** The RBC is bigger than the capillary. So the RBC needs to deform itself, ie. fold back upon itself a little bit, in order to pass through the capillary.

That's why normal RBC's are so flexible = deformable.

Bridging molecules are things that can cause RBC;s to stick together. LDL cholesterol is a bridging molecule. LDL cholesterol can get RBC's to stick together.

This briding property of LDL cholesterol is the reason why elevated LDL in the blood, causes atherosclerosis.

By the way, atherosclerosis begins as a blood clot. I'll repeat that in big red bold letters ATHEROSCLEROSIS IS A BLOOD CLOT!

That's the key to a deep understanding of atherosclerosis. Hardly any doctors know that atherosclerosis is a blood clot.

I did a fellowship in imaging guided surgery at Harvard, with the emphasis on vascular disease, and I've been studying atherosclerosis for 30 years.

The best book on atherosclerosis is the one by Gregory Sloop MD.

Anyways, the point of all this is that bridging molecules like LDL cholesterol cause the RBC's to stick together into blood sludge and rouleaux formation.

When the RBC's are stuck together, they are less deformable; ie. it's harder to push them through the capillaries.

Blood pressure must go up! Elevated blood pressure causes atherosclerosis. It's a vicious cycle. Chronic eating of a high fat diet causes chronic, relatively rapid, progressive atherosclerosis.

Atherosclerosis causes decreased oxygen delivery to tissues, and increased cancer risk.

Stress & stress equivalents cause elevated fibrinogen in the blood. Fibrinogen is a blood clotting protein. Fibrinogen is a bridging molecule. Tha's why excess stress increases the risk of rouleaux formation and related sequelae.

This is part of why learning to manage stress is part of learning how to reduce risk of cancer.

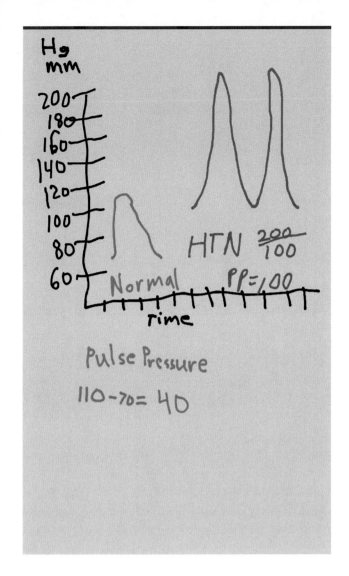

Fig 60: **Normal blood pressure is usually around 110/70** with a range of a about 90-120/60-80 depending on the individual patient.

The difference between the top number (systolic) pressure and the bottom number (diastolic) pressure is called the "pulse pressure."

High blood pressure eg. greater than 140/90 is associated with increased risk of atherosclerosis.

High blood pressure is called hypertension (HTN).

HTN damages arterial walls. Damage to arterial walls causes atherosclerosis.

Best way to prevent HTN is a low fat, low sodium, whole food, 100% vegan diet.

Plant foods are high in potassium and magnesium which are vasodilators (open up arteries).

P for Plants and P for Potassium. Magnesium is located in the center of chlorophyll, so plants are also abundant in magnesium.

Processed food is the opposite. Processed food tends to be high in sodium (vasoconstrictor), and low in potassium and magnesium.

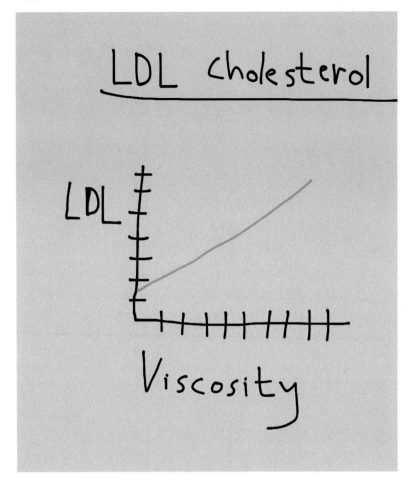

Fig 61: **Graph of LDL cholesterol vs blood viscosity.** The higher the blood LDL cholesterol, the higher the blood viscosity.

Because of increasing amounts of rouleaux formation.

The higher the blood viscosity = the thicker the blood = the higher the tendency of blood to form clots.

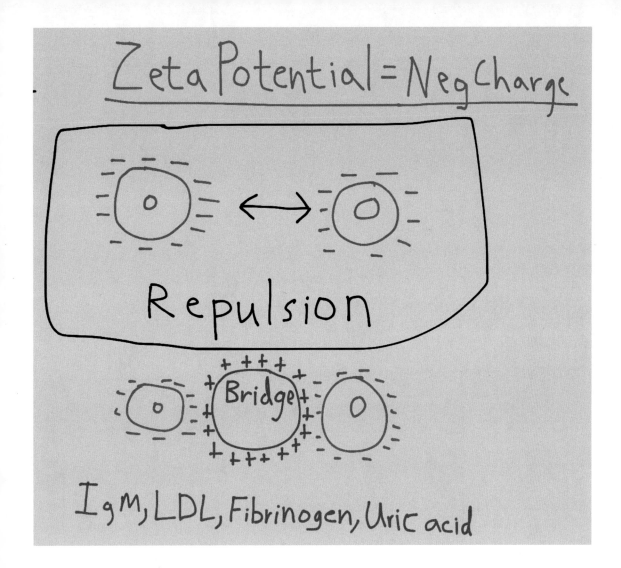

Fig 62: **RBC's have a "zeta potential."** The zeta potential is the negative charge around the outside of an RBC.

The zeta potential comes from the RBC plasma membrane-glycocalyx sialic acids, and cholesterol sulfate molecules.

The negative charge zeta potential of one RBC repels the zeta potential of adjacent RBC's. Thus, the zeta potential prevents RBC's from sticking together.

The endothelial lining also has a zeta potential, a negative charge. The zeta potential of the endothelium prevents RBC's and WBC's from sticking to the endothelium.

The WBC's also have zeta potentials, that prevent them from sticking to RBC's or the endothelium.

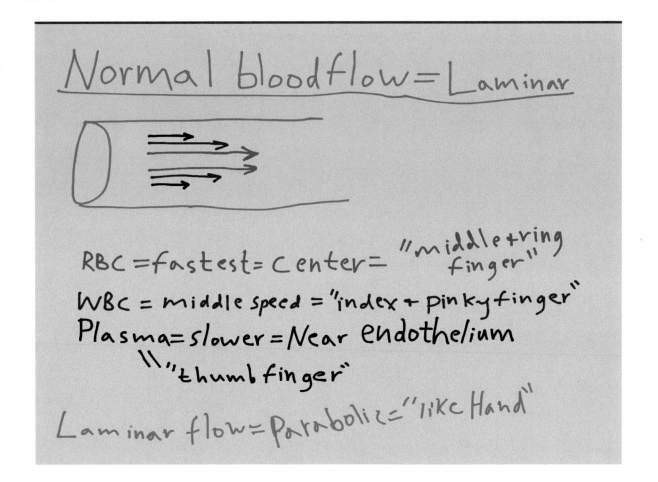

Fig 63: **Normal blood flow is laminar.** With laminar blood flow, the RBC's are in the center. WBC's are alongside the RBC's.

Plasma is in the periphery.

The arterial lining cells = endothelial cells are designed to recognize laminar flow. The like laminar flow.

Endothelial cells have mechanoreceptors that can sense, normal, laminar blood flow.

Normal blood pressure produces normal laminar blood flow.

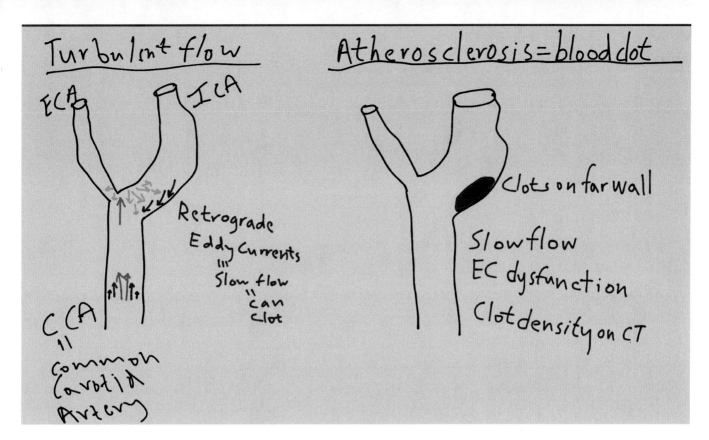

Fig 64: **Arterial bifurcations** = the site where atherosclerosis starts.

Normal blood pressure produces normal laminar blood flow.

HTN causes increased peak systolic velocity of blood flow. When the HTN related high velocity blood flow hits an arterial bifurcation, this causes turbulent blood flow, and retrograde eddy currents.

Turbulent blood flow, and retrograde eddy currents, are sensed by the endothelium as abnormal.

The endothelium sheds some of its glycocalyx ("normal sugar coating"), and prothrombotic molecules are then expressed on the endothelial surface.

Ie. the endothelium changes; instead of preventing blood clots, it starts becoming slightly pro-thrombotic (ie. clot causing).

Clot causing = atherosclerosis causing.

Atherosclerosis = decreasing oxygen delivery to tissue = increasing cancer risk.

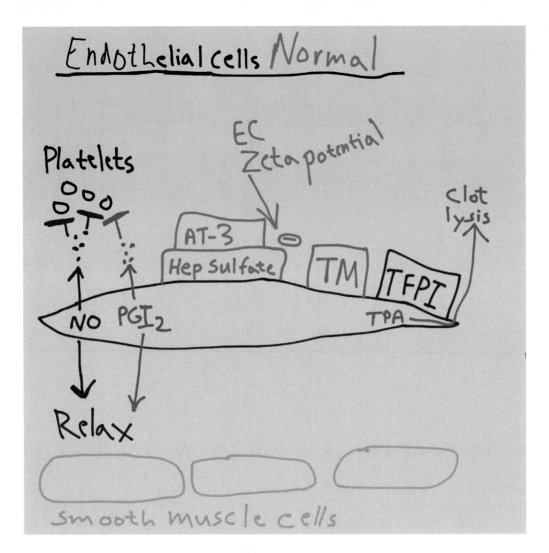

Fig 65: **Endothelial cells do a lot to prevent blood clotting.**

For endothelial cells the most important thing is that they make nitric oxide (NO). Nitroc oxide goes into the blood,and helps prevent clotting.

Nitric oxide goes into the arterial wall, and causes the smooth muscles to relax. Relaxation of arterial wall smooth walls causes vasodilation.

Vasodilation increases oxygen delivery to tissues.

It's also good to know that endothelial cells have a "glyco-calyx" = structural sugar coating.

The endothelial cell zeta potential is generated by glycocalyx sialic acids and heparan sulfates and cholesterol sulfates.

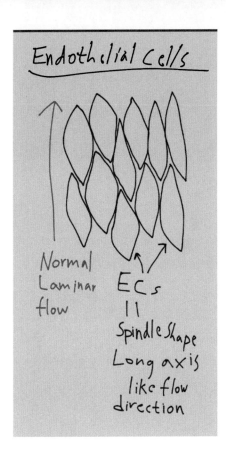

Endothelial Cells

Normal Laminar flow

ECs
||
Spindle Shape
Long axis
like flow
direction

Fig 66: **Endothelial cells typically have a spindle shape that is oriented along the direction of blood flow.**

These endothelial cells can sense if the blood is normal, ie. laminar.

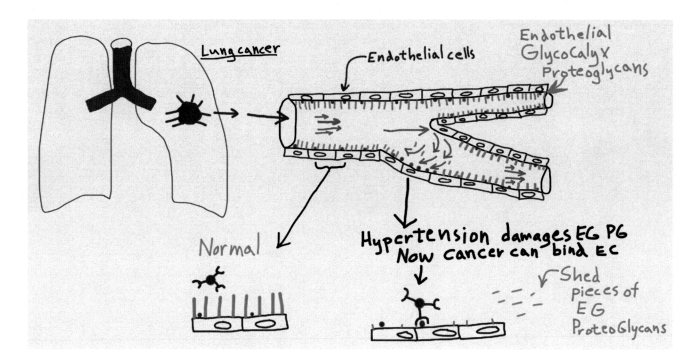

Fig 67: **Arterial bifurcations and cancer.**

When there is HTN, the endothelial cells on the far wall = away from the median divider, are the main ones to become relatively prothrombotic = adhesive.

Red blood cells for clotting, are NOT the only thing that can adhere to endothelial cells that are rendered pro-thrombotic = adhesive by HTN.

WBC's can also adhere to these abnormal, prothrombotic = adhesive endothelial cells (EC's).

From now on, I'll often abbreviate endothelial cells with EC (because the words endothelial cells comes up so often).

What's the third thing that can adhere to prothrombotic EC's?

METASTATIC CANCER CELLS!

That's one of the reasons why HTN increases the risk of cancer!

The normal EC glycocalyx is anti-thrombotic.

The abnormal EC is prothrombotic with adhesive molecules exposed on it plasma membrane.

Metastatic cancer cells can bind to the EC's and them move subintimal and become a metastatic cancer groth site.

Ref: Flow regulated endothelial glycocalyx determines metastatic cancer activity" Eno Ebong, FASEB J, 2020, May; 34 (5). Abnormal blood flow due to hypertension causes shedding of glycocalyx proteoglycans. Endothelial adhesion molecules are now exposed, and the cancer cells in the blood can bind to them.

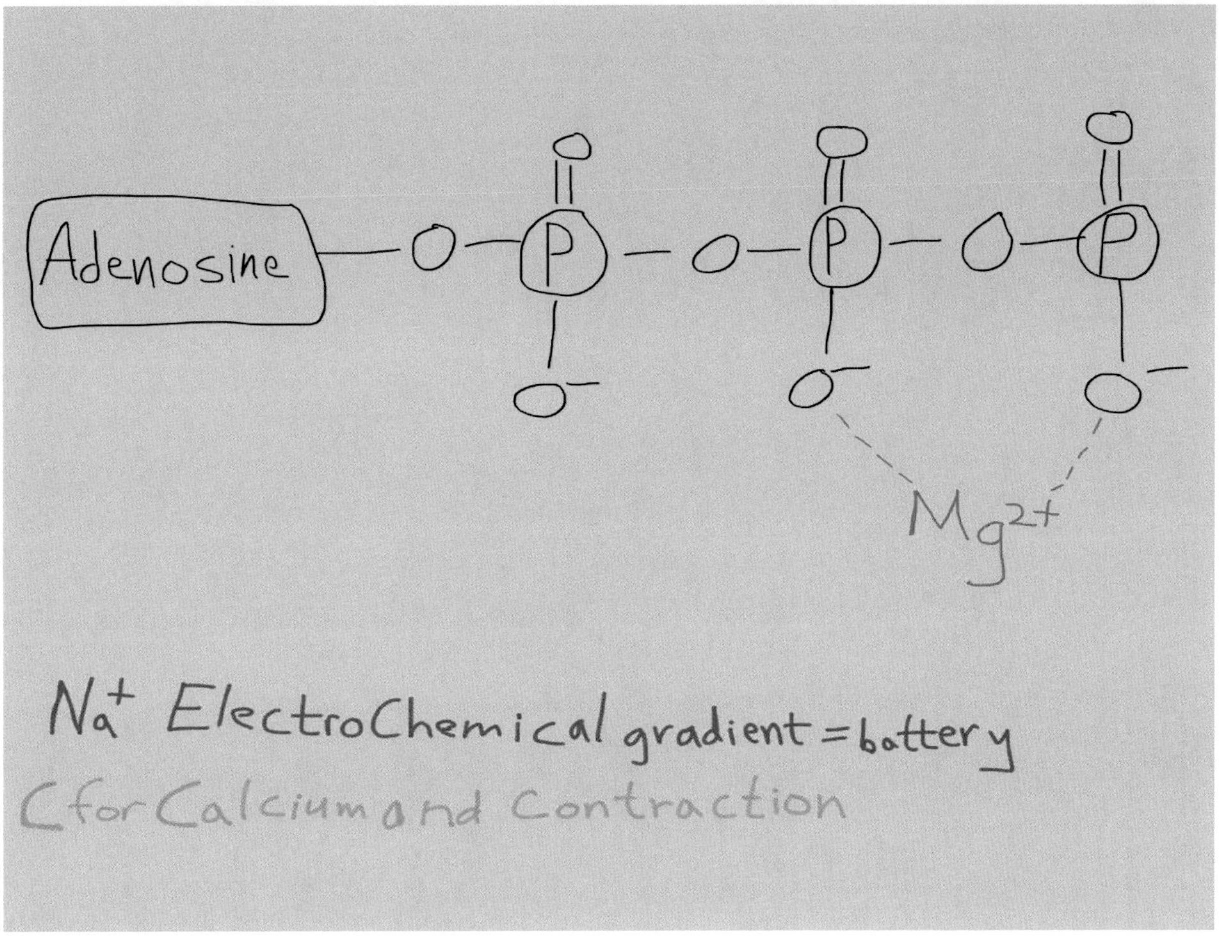

Fig 68: **Magnesium stablizes ATP.**

ATP is an Adenosine bound to Three Phosphates (A-T-P).

The phosphates have negative charges that repel each other.

The magnesium has a double positive charge = 2+.

The 2+ charge of the magnesium stablizes the ATP molecule, so that the phosphates remain stuck together.

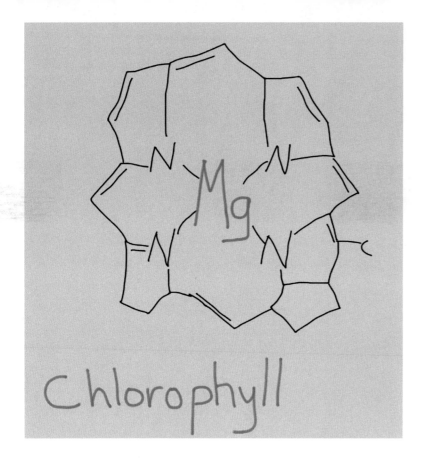

Fig 69: **Magnesium is located in the center of chlorophyll.**

Just eat plants and you will be eating chlorophyll.

"Above all, love each other deeply, for love covers over a multitude of sins. Offer hospitality to each other. Use whatever gift you have received to help others." - 1 Peter 4:8.

Above all, eat the low fat vegan diet, because it covers over a multitude of diet and lifestyle sins.

Plant diet has:

More fiber.

More potassium.

More magnesium.

More antioxidants.

More alkaline.

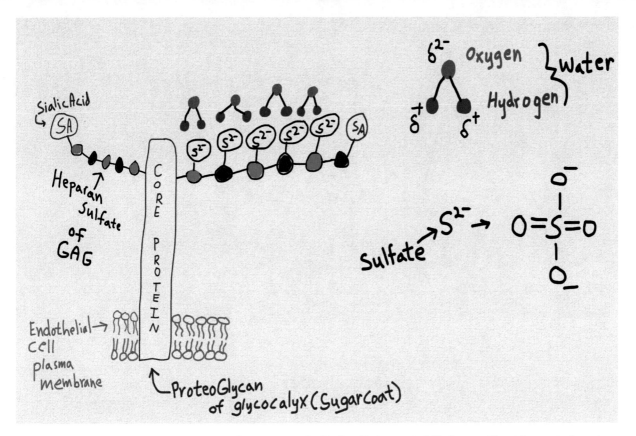

Fig 70: **Proteo-Glycan structure of the endothelial cell (arterial lining cell), Glyco-Calyx (sugar-coat).** Proteo means Protein. Glycan means Sugar. The Glycan has a polymer of sugar molecules called Heparin Sulfate.
Sorry for all the jargon, but it's good to know about the **endothelial cell (EC) glycocalyx (GC).**

The polymer (polymer means chain of) sugar molecules is called a **GAG (Glycos-Amino-Glycan).**

At the end tip of the GAG is a **Sialic Acid (SA).**

What's the point? The GAG & the SA have a negative charge. That's a lot of negative charge!

Why does it have so much negative charge? Because it generates a **ZETA POTENTIAL!**

Ie. the endothelial cell – like RBC's & WBC's – also has a zeta potential = a negative charge on its outer surface.

Why do they all have zeta potentials? So that they don't stick together = so that they don't clot!

The **endothelial cell (EC)** glycocalyx zeta potential attracts water, because water is charged.

The hydrogens have a partial positive charge which is attracted to the negative charge of the EC glycocalyx.

The EC glycocalyx has the consistency of jello. This jello = gel consistency covered with water is "slippery."

I'm sure you've heard the expression "slippery when wet."

Why did God make the EC glycocalyx so slippery? So that RBC's and WBC's can more easily pass through the arteries and veins and NOT stick to the walls!

It's a brilliant system. It works great for life if a person eats plant foods. Yanomamo, Tarahumara, rural Kenyans and other plant eating populations have normal blood pressures all their lives.

It's the meat & oils of processed foods that messes up the RBC's and the arterial walls & causes hypertension, diabetes, and atherosclerosis.

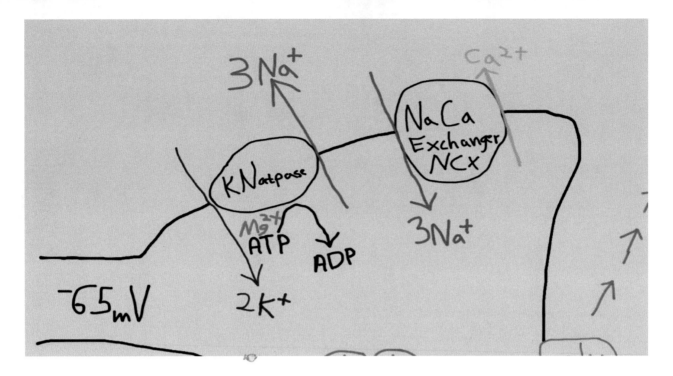

Fig 71: **Potassium = K+, Sodium = Na+ ATPase pump = KN Atpase = KNA.** The plasma membrane of all human cells has a Potassium, Sodium pump. The plasma membrane of a cell is the outer membrane of the cell.

The potassium sodium pump requires ATP for energy, so it is called ACTIVE transport. K stands for Kalium = latin word for potassium. N stands for Na which stands for Natrium = latin word for sodium.

I like to put the "K" first in the name, to indicate that K+ is pumped INTO the cell.

How much cell energy is used for the KNA? Many cells use 1/3 of their ATP for KNA. Neurons use 2/3 of their energy for KNA!

That's a lot of energy!

Why would a cell use so much energy for the KNA? Because, KNA maintains an electric and chemical gradient across the plasma cell membrane. KNA is a battery!

KNA converts the ATP into an all purpose energy source for pumping things into and out of the cell. That's what cells need to do = take in good stuff like food, and pump out bad stuff like waste products.

To run KNA optimally, the person needs to eat "normal" amounts of potassium & sodium.

Humans are designed by God to normally eat a lot more potassium than sodium.

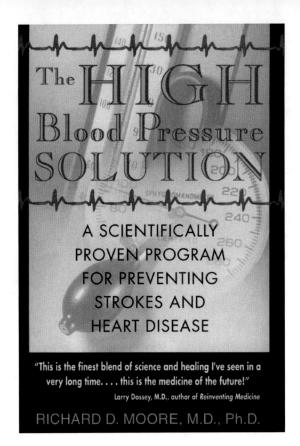

Fig 72: **The High blood pressure solution by Richard Moore, MD, Phd** is the best book ever written about blood pressure. It's one of the best medical books ever written. It's a masterpiece.

According to Richard Moore, who devoted his entire life to researching KNA, he says humans need to eat at least 5x more potassium than sodium.

He says that a person needs to eat 5x more potassium than sodium if they want to prevent hypertension.

Our ancestors probably ate about 25x more potassium than sodium.

Where does potassium come from? P for Potassium and P for plants.

Richard Moore says that we also need to eat adequate amounts of magnesium, because the magnesium is needed to stabilize ATP.

Where does magnesium come from? Magnesium is located smack dab in the center of chlorophyll.

Where does chlorophyll come from? Chlorophyll is THE molecule of photosynthesis = plants!

Who has to be careful about eating large amounts of potassium? Patients with severe kidney failure, (a very small part of the population), might need to reduce their intake of potassium, because normally the kidney excrete excess dietary potassium.

Patients with kidney failure should consult their doctors before changing their diets.

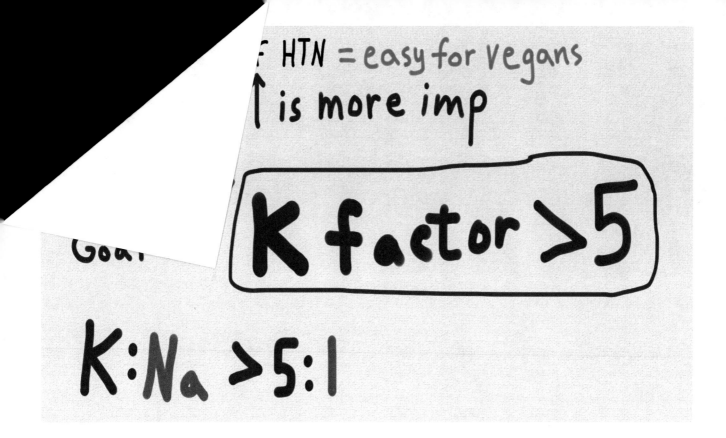

Fig 73: **K factor is the ratio of dietary K to Na.** Richard Moore recommends K factor > 5, at least.

K factor is the secret of hypertension that doctors don't know. K+ > Na+.

I never count or measure my potassium intake. I just eat plant foods, and the body takes care of everything else.

I probably eat a K factor of about 25:1, just like our ancestors did, because I am a 100% whole food vegan.

That's the great secret of health: to live like Adam & Eve, but to keep modern indoor heating and plumbing.

When you eat the foods that we are designed to eat, your cells function better.

Better cell function helps you to avoid hypertension and atherosclerosis and diabetes = to reduce risk of obesity, impotence, heart disease and cancer!

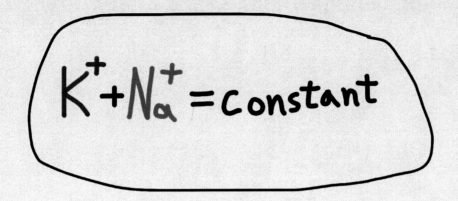

To maintain osmolality + mbr voltage inside cell

$$K^+ + Na^+ = constant$$

Fig 74: **The KN constant.** The human body MUST maintain a fixed amount of positively charged ions in the extracellular space and inside of cells.

Positively charged ions are called "CAT- ions." You can remember "P"ositively charged by a cat "P"urrs, and a carnivore cat likes to lick salt.

The human body MUST maintain a fixed amount of positively charged ions in the extracellular space and inside of cells.

When a person eats excess sodium – as most Americans do – the body automatically starts pissing out potassium.

The body has to reduce its quantity of cations.

What's the point? When a person eats too much sodium, they piss out their potassium; and this messes up their plasma membrane gradients!

When the plasma membrane gradients of sodium and potassium ions are messed up, then the KNA pumps do not work so well.

Then the cell has difficulty pumping other things like calcium ions.

Potassium and sodium ions are the minimum wage worker ions of the cell who do all the manual labor.

Calcium is the aristocrat ion of the cell. When Calcium enters the cell it starts bossing everybody around, and making things happen.

Calcium entry makes big events happen.

When calcium enters a muscle cell, it CONTRACTS.

When calcium enters a neuron (brain cell) it FIRES an ACTION POTENTIAL.

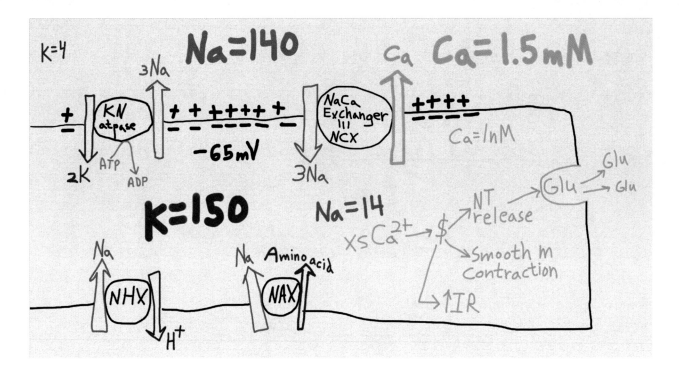

Fig 75: **How the plasma membrane does work.** KN Atpase maintains an ELECTRICAL gradient of about -65 millivolts = -65 mV.

KNA also maintains a sodium CONCENTRATION gradient with sodium concentration outside the cell of 140, and inside the cell of 14.

That's a sodium gradient of 10x more sodium outside the cell, than inside the cell.

Sodium wants to equalize its concentration gradient. Sodium WANTS to go into the cell!

When an ion travels along its concentration gradient, it's movement generates energy.

This energy is coupled to other jobs of the cell.

The energy of sodium entry is coupled to pumping out potassium at the NaCa exchanger. Na stands for sodium. Ca stands for calcium.

NaCa exchanger is often abbreviated NCX.

Cells need the NCX to be able to pump out calcium ions quickly.

Sodium ions = Na ions are also coupled to pumping out protons = H+, and to pumping in amino acids.

The energy for the majority of work done inside a cell comes from ATP and KNA.

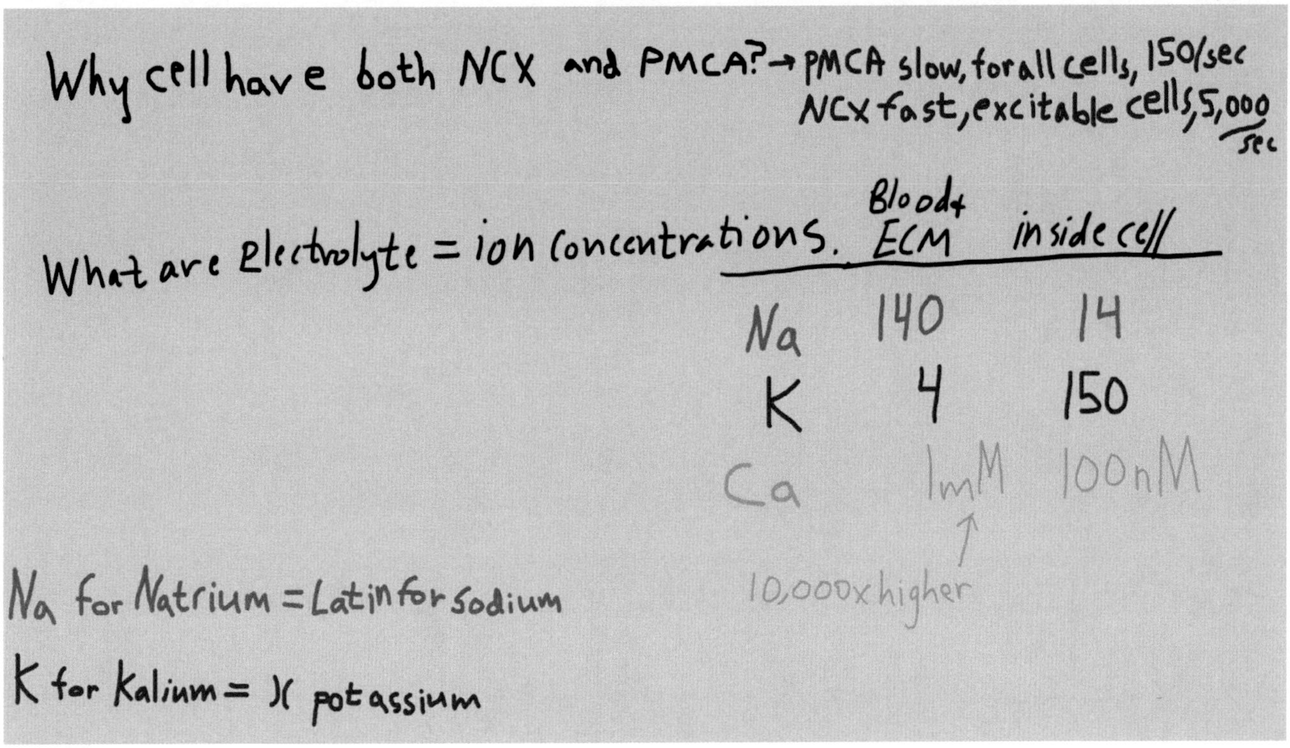

Why cell have both NCX and PMCA? → PMCA slow, for all cells, 150/sec

NCX fast, excitable cells, 5,000/sec

What are electrolyte = ion concentrations.

	Blood+ ECM	inside cell
Na	140	14
K	4	150
Ca	$1mM$	$100nM$

10,000x higher

Na for Natrium = Latin for sodium

K for Kalium =)(potassium

Fig 76: **Ion concentrations in the extracellular matrix and inside cells.**

Notice that sodium = Na is 10x higher outside the cell, than inside the cell.

Notice that calcium = Ca is 10,000x higher outside the cell than inside the cell.

Sodium really wants to go into the cell.

Calcium really, really, really, really wants to go into the cell.

For folks who want to get technical, the KNA pumps 2 potassium into of the cell for every 3 sodiums that are pumped out.

I sometimes abbreviate it like this: K_2N_3A.

Because more positive charges are pumped out = 3 sodiums, than positive charges pumped in = 2 potassiums, this makes the charge inside the cell more negative.

Because ATP is used by the KNA, the KNA is called "primary active transport."

When the sodium electrochemical gradient is used to pump other things, like Calcium, that is called "secondary active transport."

Bottom line: A healthy K factor helps your cells to function better & helps prevent hypertension.

Cells that are functioning well are much less likely to develop cancer.

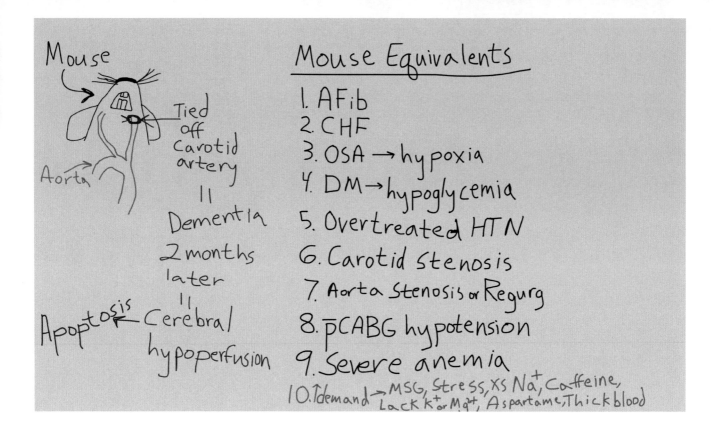

Figure 77: **The Jack de la Torre theory of dementia.**

The carotid artery is the main blood flow to the brain. There is one carotid artery on each side of the neck.

Jack de la Torre Phd is a scientist who tied off the carotid artery in the neck of a mouse. De la Torre expected the mouse to have a big stroke. (Stroke is when an artery in the brain is occluded and this kills brain cells suddenly due to the anoxia (lack of oxygen).

After tying off the carotic artery in the neck of the mouse, on one side, de la Torre (dlT) noticed that mouse typicaly became demented two months later.

DlT decided to do an autopsy. When he cracked open the little mouse skull, he expected to see a big stroke… but there was no stroke.

What happened to the mouse brain? How come there was no stroke? What did dlT actually see?

On the side the carotid artery had been tied off, the mouse brain was shrunken. The medical word for shrunken is "atrophic."

The medical word for "same" is "ipsi. The medical word for "side" is "lateral." The ispi-lateral mouse brain = same side as carotid artery had been tied off.

Why was the ispilateral brain atrophic (smaller, but otherwise looks normal) rather than stroked out (necrotic, dead, destroyed)?

Because some blood was still getting to the ipsilateral mouse brain from the other arteries that supply the brain like the carotid artery on the other side of the neck, and the vertebral arteries in the back of the brain.

So, the ispilateral brain was GRADUALLY losing brain cells via apoptosis (slow cell death = programmed cell death = from hypoxia (partial oxygen loss) rather than anoxia (total oxygen loss).

Well so what? What does dlT's mice have to do with dementia?

How many Americans do you know over 50 years of age who are hypertensive? The majority of them!

Why are they hypertensive? Usually because they eat too much fat which makes their blood thick, and too much sodium and caffeine which constricts their arteries, and this increases blood pressure.

Also, they are fat, and the heart needs to generate more pressure to pump blood to a big fat body, rather than a smaller, skinny body.

Why does the body raise blood pressure? Where is the most difficult place to pump blood?

To get blood to the brain! The top of the brain is the greatest distance from the heart that is against gravity!

When the ADS (Average Dumb Shit) realizes they are hypertensive, what do they do? They go to a doctor.

What does the doctor do? He looks at a chart of medical recommendations for blood pressure treatment.

Why is blood pressure treated with pills?

Because of blood pressure goes to high, it can cause a stroke; very high blood pressure also damages other organs like the eyes and the kidneys; and severe hypertension (HTN) causes atherosclerosis everywhere.

Okay, so what's the point? What happens when the pills reduce blood pressure too much?

Don't you know it's rude to answer a question with a question?!

Yes, of course, but sometimes a question to a question is the best answer. A rhetorical question focuses attention in a new way.

If the pill lowers blood pressure too much, it becomes a **MOUSE EQUIVALENT!!!!!!**

Millions of ADS's are overtreating their HTN & potentially going to end up demented like the mouse, with atrophic brains.

De la Torre said that any cause of chronic cerebral hypopersfusion could make the mice demented.

There are lots of causes of chronic cerebral hypoperfusion like aortic regurgitation, aortic stenosis, atrial fibrillation, post surgical hypotension, etc.

What does this have to do with preventing cancer? Chronic hypoperfusion of an organ causes tissue hypoxia; tissue hypoxia increases the risk of cancer. Healthy brain enables you to make smarter choices for restoring your health.

What about the Peter Rogers MD theory of dementia due to neuro-vascular uncoupling? That theory explains how most people damage their brains by ingesting multiple, simultaneous neuro-toxic chemicals in addition to excess dietary fat and sodium.

How about some examples of other neurotoxic chemicals?

Hexane often used to process soy.
Caffeine = cerebral artery vasoconstrictor and stimulant (excitotoxin)
Fluoride in tap water, toothpaste, mouthwash, POFA cookware, many medications.
Aluminum in tap water, and cans and cookware.
MSG (MonoSodium Glutamate) and Mfg (Manufactured free Glutamate).
Gly-phosphate (a probable excitotoxin)
Aspartame (excitotoxin)
High Fructose Corn Syrup (HFCS) contaminated with mercury.
Omega 6 fats leading to HNE (HydroxyNonEnal) inhibits mitochondria
Other mitochondrial inhibitors like TCE (TriChloroEthylene), lead, cadmium
SERCA (Sarcoplasm Endoplasmic Reticulum) Calcium ATPase inhibitors like BHA, BHT, etc.

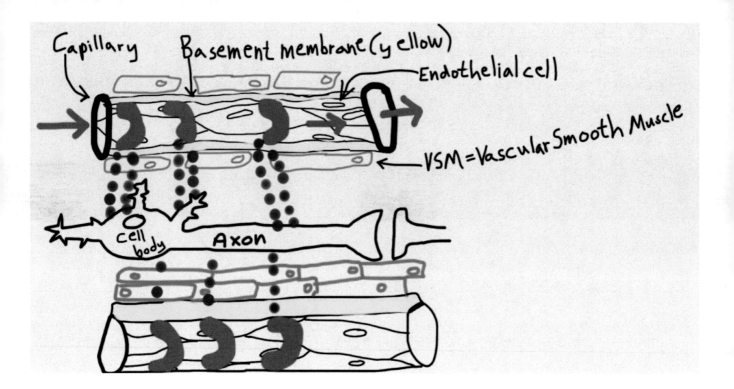

Fig 78: **Normal capillaries versus capillaries with diabetes and hypertension.** The RBC's are in red. The black circles are the capillary entrance and exit. The yellow stripe is the capillary basement membrane.

The spindle shaped cells are the endothelial cells (note how they are aligned along the long axis of the direction of blood flow).

The green cells are the vascular smooth cells (and there are more in this drawing than is usually present for the purpose of conveying vascular smooth muscle hypertrophy in hypertension).

The blue circles are oxygen.

The normal capillary enables LOTS of OXYGEN to travel to the tissue (which in this case is a neuron).

The lower capillary is diseased by diabetes and hypertension. The lower capillary is characteristic of most middle age and older Americans.

Notice that less oxygen travels from the diseased capillary.

Notice that the diabetes and hypertension have caused the capillary basement membrane to become thickened;

Notice that the diabetes and hypertension have caused the vascular smooth muscle cells to become bigger (hypertrophy) and more numerous (hyperplasia).

Notice that the diseased capillary has a thicker wall than the normal capillary.

The diseased capillary contributes to decreasing oxygen delivery to the tissues.

Decreased oxygen delivery is called hypoxia.

Hypoxia increases risk of cancer causation and cancer growth!

Therefore, preventing diabetes and HTN helps to prevent cancer!

What prevents diabetes and HTN? The same things that prevent most diseases = low fat, low sodium, 100% vegan, whole food, with no sweets, no caffeine, no oil, no alcohol, no tobacco, etc.

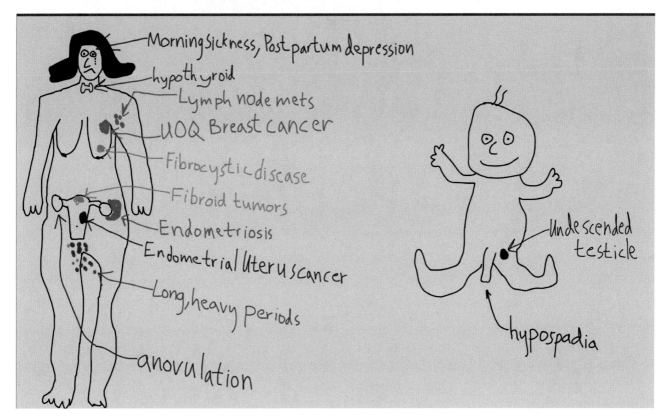

Fig 79: **Estrogen overload effects.**

Excess estrogen and estrogenic chemicals can cause:

- Heavy menstrual periods

- PMS = Pre Menstrual Syndrome

- Uterine fibroids (benign tumors)

- Anovulation = infertility (estrogenic chemical EE2 is a common contraceptive)

- Breast cancer

- Congenital birth defects in boys (like hypospadias and undescended testicle) and girls

- Increased risk of autoimmune disease

- Increased breasts fibrocystic disease

- **Increased risk of breast cancer**

- **Increased risk of uterine cancer = endometrial cancer**

- **Increased risk of protate cancer**

- Postmenopausal hot flashes

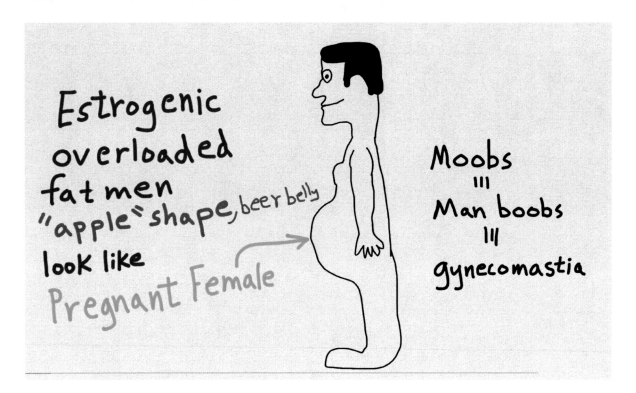

Fig 80: **The estrogen overloaded man.** His man boobs (moobs) are not just fat; they may also contain hypertrophied breast ductal cells (that's called gyne-co-mastia = female like breasts).

His big bell is due to fat, but it certainly resembles a pregnant female. Many often call the big fat male belly a "beer belly" or an "apple shape," but lets be honest.

He looks like a pregnant female.

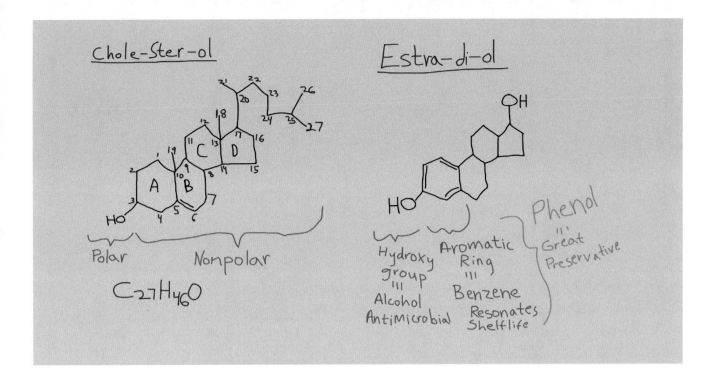

Fig 81: Cholesterol and Estrogen chemical structures. Cholesterol has 4 cyclic rings. Ring A, carbon #3 is attached to a hydroxyl group which is also called an alcohol group and represented by "-OH."

In cholester-ol, the ol at the end of the word stands for alcoh-ol group.

All the sex hormones are built on the cyclic rings of cholesterol.

Estradiol is an estrogen.

Estra-di-ol has two alcohol groups.

The most important features of estradiol are that ring A now has 3 double bonds. When a 6 carbon ring has 3 double bonds, it is called an aromatic (because it smells) or a benzene.

Because of the benzene ring, many estrogenic chemicals will include the prefix "benzyl."

The 3 double bonds make the 6 carbon ring much more stable; ie. in chemistry "stable" means less likely to change = longer shelf life.

The hydroxyl (or alcohol) group attached to the aromatic ring has antimicrobial properties (it kills mold).

Can you see how estrogenic chemicals are great for preservatives?

The aromatic ring confers a long shelf life stability.

The hydroxyl group confers anti-mold properties.

That's why estrogenic preservatives are in almost all personal care products.

By the way, the combination of an aromatic ring plus a hydroxyl group is called a "phenol" group.

That name "phenol" and its prefix "phenyl" will come up a lot with estrogenic chemicals.

In fact, if you are ever reading the ingredients list on a food or a personal care product and it says "benzyl" or "phenyl," you can reasonably assume it's an estrogenic chemical.

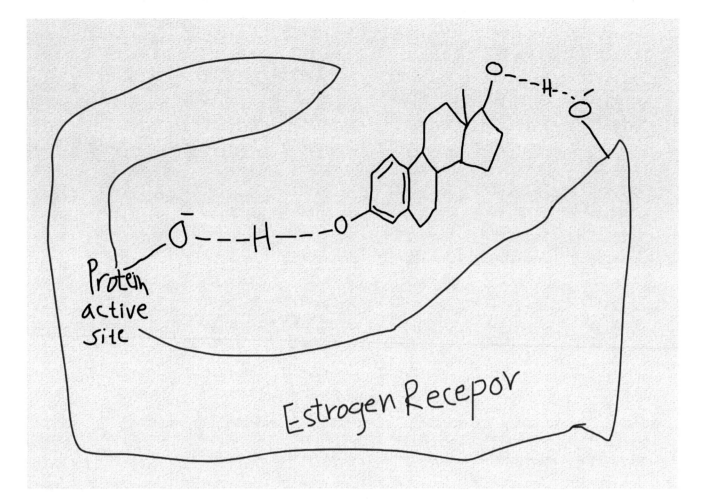

Fig 82: **Estrogen interacting with the estrogen receptor.**

Estrogen or an estrogenic chemical binds to the estrogen receptor, and the estrogen receptor then initiates estrogenic hormonal effects.

The hydroxyl group on the aromatic ring is what forms a hydrogen bond with the estrogen receptor.

Evolutionarily the estrogen molecule didn't really have any competition.

This led to the estrogen receptor becoming "lazy," "not too fussy," a bit of a "promiscuous whore in the modern world."

What am I saying?

Any molecule with an aromatic ring in the corner, that's attached to a hydroxyl group can potentially bind the estrogen receptor.

There's a lot of molecules like that!

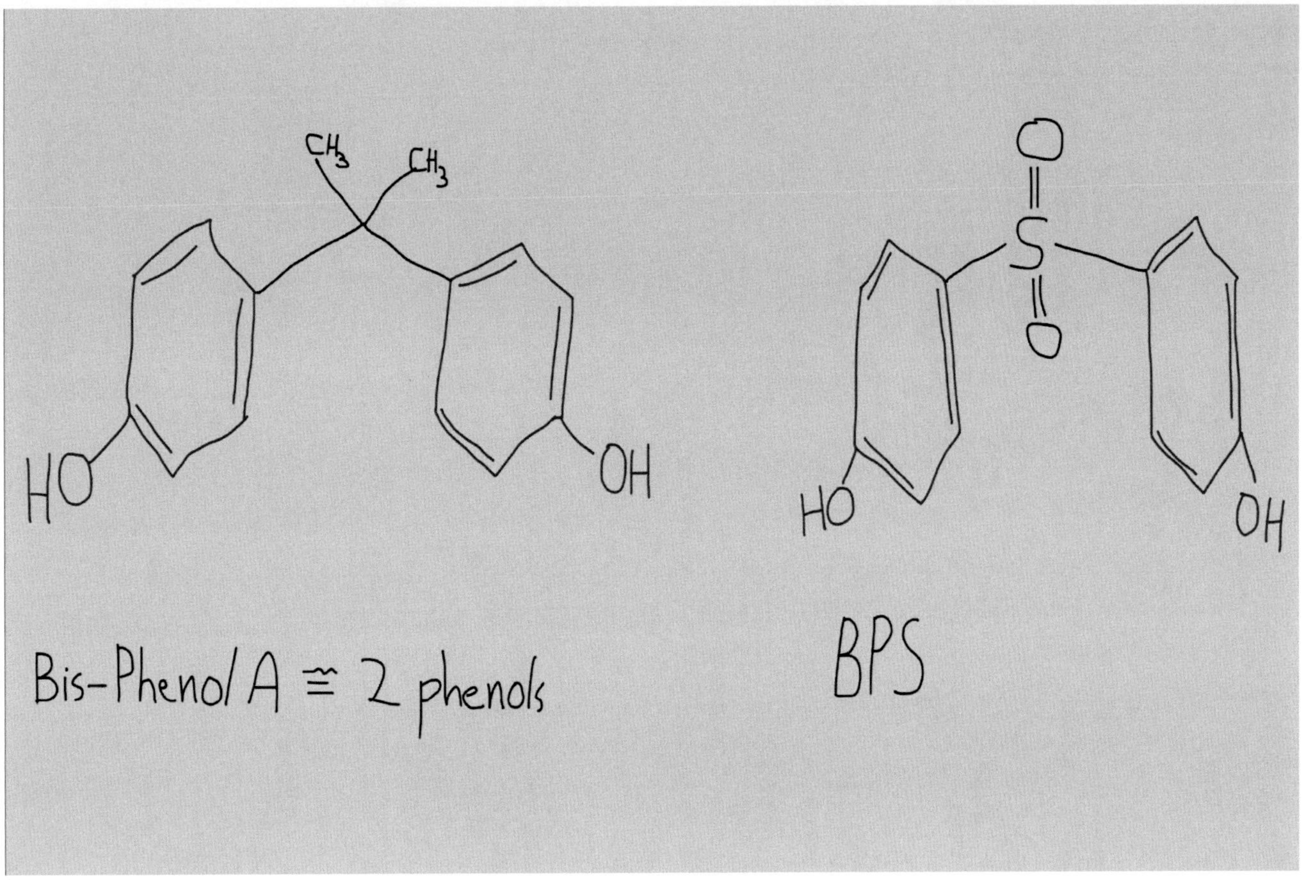

Bis-Phenol A ≅ 2 phenols   BPS

Fig 83: **BPA is Bis Phenol A.** In chemistry, Bis means two of the same things. Bis in BPA means 2 phenol groups.

A phenol group is an aromatic ring and a hydroxyl group.

Notice that BPA has a phenol group on both sides.

Remember that the hydroxyl group binds with the estrogen receptor.

BPA is very common in plastics.

BPA containers, eg. for bottled water, leach into the water.

Many people got upset about BPA leaching intot he water and other beverages so they demanded that BPA be banned.

The food companies just laughed. "Sure," they said.

The food companies can easily just substitute the middle of the molecule with something else, and make a related molecule, like BPS.

The BPS in the above figure still has 2 phenol groups, and will exert an estrogenic effect.

That's why water should be stored in glass, and not plastic.

BPA or BPA equivalents are used in many plastics, and this puts the person who uses these things at risk for BPA exposure.

You can't completely avoid being exposed to BPA and BPA like chemicals, but you can minimize the amount of exposure.

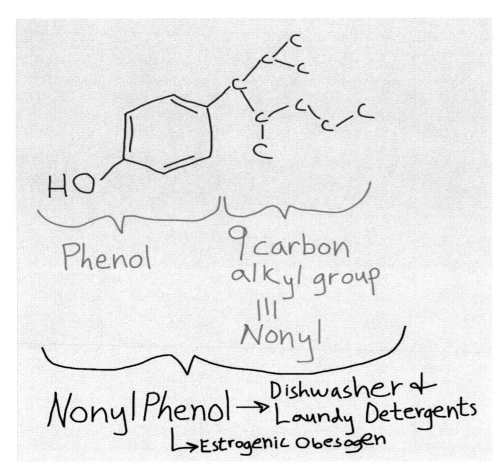

Fig 84: **Nonyl-Phenol is used for dishwasher and laundry detergents.** Non means nine = for the nine carbon side chain.

Phenol means phenol for the estrogenic component.

If you don't cook with oils, then you don't need to use a dish washer, and then don't need dish washing detergent.

For my laundry, I just wash the clothes in hot water with no detergent.

This is how I avoid estrogenic chemicals.

I just rinse my hair with water. I do not use shampoo. The typical shampoo has 2 or 3 estrogenic chemicals.

Being a minimalist enables you to save money and avoid estrogenics.

The only chemical in my bathroom is one bar of transparent soap (with the fewest chemicals possible).

For comparison, in my wife's bathroom, she has 55 personal care products.

I told her that she was stupid; that she was rubbing estrogenic chemicals on herself.

Wife: You don't understand! A woman would rub shit on her face, if she thought it would make her more pretty.

Me: Well that's basically what you are doing.

Wife: You're just jealous, because you have more wrinkles than me. Right in the center of your forehead, you have a big "bitch" line. A really BIG bitch line!

She was a cosmetologist before she became a doctor, so she thinks her wrinkle creams are slowing down aging. She also does cosmetic injection procedures, and whenever I annoy her, she tells me I have big "bitch" lines on my face.

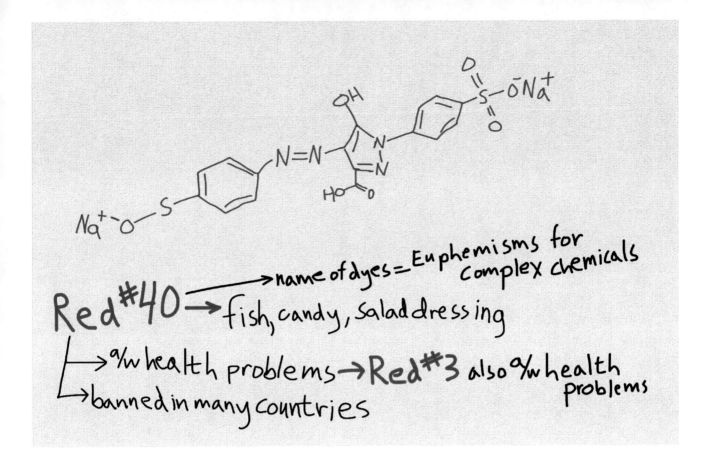

Red#40 → name of dyes = Euphemisms for complex chemicals
→ fish, candy, Salad dressing
↳ %w health problems → Red#3 also %w health problems
↳ banned in many Countries

Fig 85: **Red dye #40 has estrogenic properties.**

BenzoPhenone

(Aromatic ketone)

DiPhenyl Methanone

OxyBenzophenone (OBP)
|||
BenzoPhenone 3 → BP3 → Sunscreen (very common)
|||
UVfilter → EDC, absorbs into blood 8% → Toxic to Coral + Marine life, often banned
↳ a/w Endometriosis

Fig 86: **Some chemicals in sunscreens like oxyBENZOphenone or BENZOphenone 3 are estrogenic.**

I made videos at you tube channel "Peter Rogers MD" about estrogenic chemicals and about sunscreens.

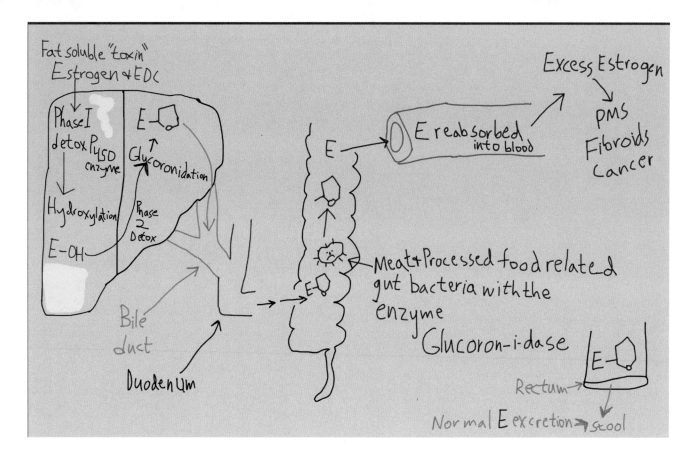

Fig 87: **Estrogen excretion from the human body.**

The liver detoxifies chemicals typically by making them more polar = adding hyroxyl groups and other polar groups, like glucoronic acid.

The chemical is then excreted into the bile, or the chemical may reenter the blood, and then travel to the kidney, and be excreted by the kidney.

The liver is part of the immune system. The liver helps remove many toxic chemicals from the body.

During phase one of detoxification, the liver adds a hydroxyl group to the molecule, to make it more polar (more charged, more soluble in water, blood, bile, urine).

During phase 2 deotoxification, the liver adds an even more polar molecule, like glucoronic acid. Adding a glucoronic acid is called "conjugation."

When estrogen levels in the blood are high, the liver takes the estrogen, and puts it through phase 1 and phase 2 detoxification.

The liver then excretes the conjugated estrogen into the bile.

Normally, the person defecates the conjugated estrogen to get it out of the body.

However, when a person eats meat and oils, those foods lack fiber. The lack of fiber leads to a different gut bacterial microbiome.

The meat and oil related gut bacteria have an excess of the enzyme called "glucoronidase." The bad bacteria glucoronidase breaks the bond between estrogen and glucoronic acid.

When estrogen is free of the glucoronic acid, then the gut will absorb it, back into the blood.

What's the point? Persons who eat meat and oils have bad bacteria in their gut; these bad bacteria have more of the enzyme glucoronidase; they end up reabsorbing estrogen; they have high body levels of estrogen; they have high risk of estrogenic cancers like breast cancer, uterine cancer and prostate cancer.

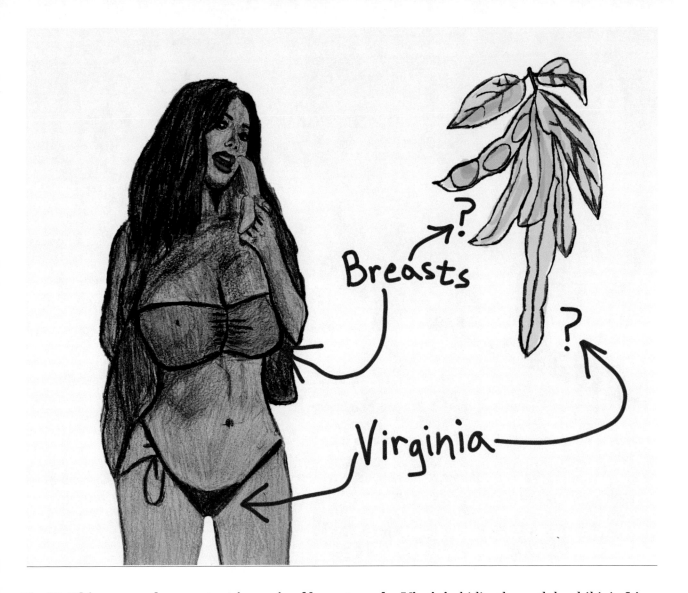

Fig 88: **This woman has an amazing pair of breasts and a Virginia** hiding beneath her bikini. It's OBVIOUS why she has high estrogen level.

She puts that estrogen to good use. She can please a man, and make a baby.

The real question is why does that soy plant have such high estrogenic chemicals.

The soy plant does NOT have any breasts. The soy plant does NOT have a Virginia.

High levels of estrogenic chemicals can cause anovulation and infertility. Maybe soy is trying to kill off the animals that eat it by making them infertile.

Soy estrogens are called phyto-estrogens.

Soy estrogens do activate both the alpha and the beta estrogen receptors.

I go into far more detail about the problems associated with soy on the videos at my you tube channel.

I know that a lot of people claim that soy is a "healthy food."

My extensive study of the scientific literature suggests that it is a harmful food, and should be avoided.

Soy is often processed with hexane = a neurotoxin.

Soy is associated with increased risk of hypothyroidism.

The herbicide gly-phosphate that is sprayed on soy has multiple potential harmful effects.

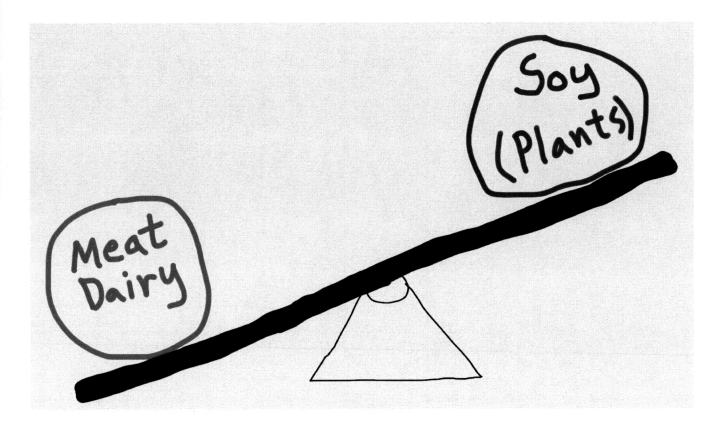

Fig 89: **Why do so many people think soy is a health food?**

When people change from a meat, dairy and oils diet to a vegetarian or vegan diet, they often stop eating meat, dairy and oils, and replace it with plants and soy.

The person gets LOTS of benefits by quitting the meat, dairy and oils.

The person, and the researchers often wrongly think the benefits came from soy.

The soy making companies put out many bogus papers that exaggerate any theoretical "benefits" of soy.

How can I be so sure?

When you look at the older papers, written before there was financial interest in soy, one sees LOTS of problems with soy.

Also the modern researchers find lots of problems with soy. It just takes more effort to find the negative information on soy, than the positive, and few people make the effort.

There are also a lot of liars on the internet who are trying to promote soy and make bogus claims about it.

If you want, you can see my online videos on soy where I go through many of the scientific papers showing problems with soy.

Dr Anthony Jay Phd, a lipid biochemist has made online videos about soy; and he wrote an excellent book called "Estrogeneration" that talks about the problems with soy.

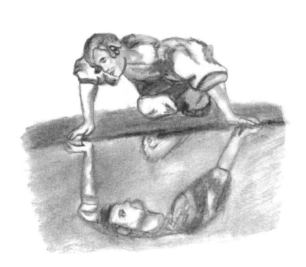

Fig 90: **Problems with the vegan diet.**

Most common side effect of vegan diet is that you become so thin and energetic that you fall in love with yourself again; and start spending too much time in front of mirrors.

The first week or two, you might get the "farts," because good gut bacteria are replacing the old "half ass" gut bacteria.

Another side effect of becoming a vegan is increased energy levels. It's common that a person wants to exercise more.

Many newly converted vegans start running distance races, or even become marathoners or triatheletes; eg. Garth Davis MD, bariatric surgeon, who became a triathlete.

Garth Davis also wrote a good book called "protein-a-holic" explaining some of the problems with a high protein diet.

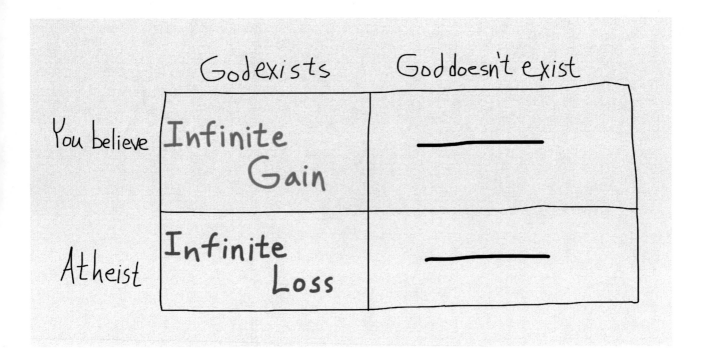

Fig 91: **Pascal's wager with religion and health.**

Religious people are healthier. Believing that life has meaning is more inspiring than believing it doesn't.

Believing that humans are created in the image of God leads to much better societies than atheism.

If you look at history, you will see most of mankind's greatest achievements were created by religious people.

Best painter and sculptor = Michelangelo = painted Sistine chapel ceiling and wall = devout Catholic.

Best illustrator = Raphael = painted the School of Athens = Catholic

Great Victorian age painters = Pre-Raphaelite brotherhood = John Everett Millais, Edmund Leighton, etc = Christians

Best architecture = French Cathedrals like Notre Dame, Chartre = devout Catholic

Best novels = Christmas Carol by Charles Dickens, Les Miserables by Victor Hugo, Brothers Karamazov by Fyodor Dostoevsky = all are Christians, and all these books with Christian themes.

Invention of the modern scientific method = Catholics.

Inventor of the modern university = Catholics

Best scientist who ever lived = Isaac Newton = devout Protestant Christian.

Best music = Bach, Handel, Mozart, Beethoven, Chopin, Schubert, etc = Christian.

Religion energizes people.

In national geographic researcher, Dan Beuttner's book, "Blue Zones" about the five longest lived, healthiest populations in the world, they all were religious.

Seventh Day Adventist vegans in Loma Linda California of USA were the longest lived population in the world.

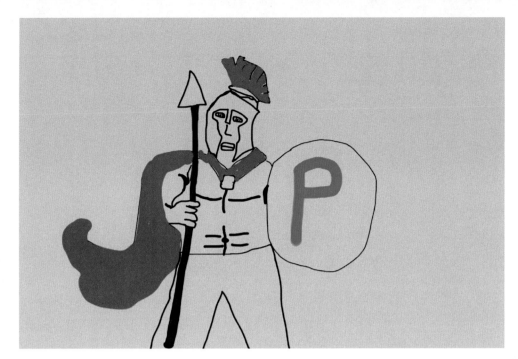

Fig 92: **Spartan Vegan diet = only starches, fruits, veggies & vitamin B12.**

It's simple, cheap & effective. Spartan calls to mind the ancient Greek Spartans who were strong; and my previous life as a wrestler.

Spartan also calls to mind keeping it simple; easy to learn; easy to do.

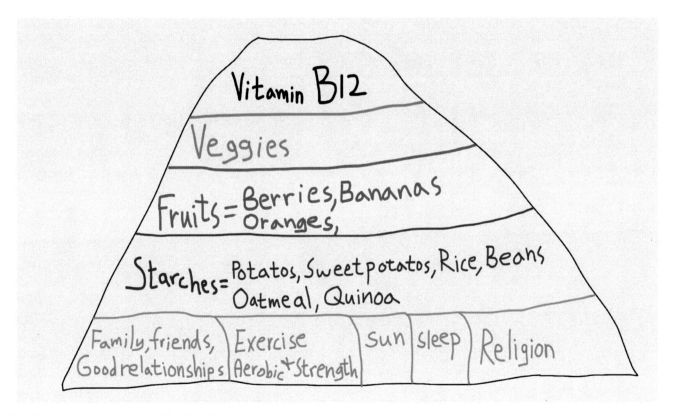

Fig 93: **Spartan Vegan diet food pyramid.**

The lifestyle stuff in the bottom row is easy to learn and a pleasure.

Starches are easy to cook. You just boil them. All of them. Starches are cheap. Starches are easy to store. Starches are the best food to satisfy hunger. Starches satisfy hunger with the fewest calories.

Fruits taste great, but are less filling than starches. Fruits are more expensive. Fruits last longer with refridgeration or freezing.

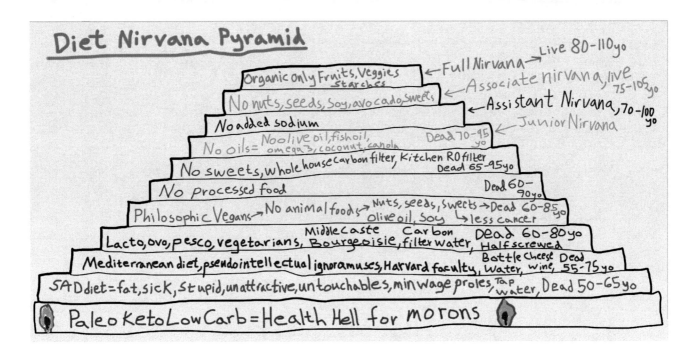

Fig 94: **A fancier version of a food pyramid called diet nirvana pyramid** with comparison of diets.

Spartan vegan diet = full nirvana.

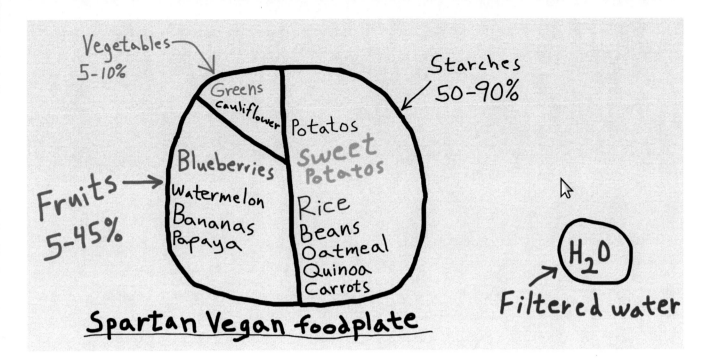

Fig 95: **Spartan Vegan foodplate.**

Only eat good foods, and do not eat bad foods.

Good foods are starches, fruits and vegetables.

Do not drink tap water. Water should be filtered.

I have a well water with a whole house carbon filter and a kitchen reverse osmosis (RO) filter.

I think that RO water tends to be a little bit "over purified" in the sense that it can have a very low TDS (Total Dissolved Solids);

which can make it hypo-osmolar. To drink hypo-osmolar water alone can cause headaches, etc in some people.

I would never drink RO water alone, without eating a decent amount first, to get some "osmotic" particles into my stomach and blood first.

I seldom drink water, unless it is to chase down food. If I were to drink RO water, I would do something like squeeze a lemon into it first to increase osmolality.

I would always eat first, before drinking RO water.

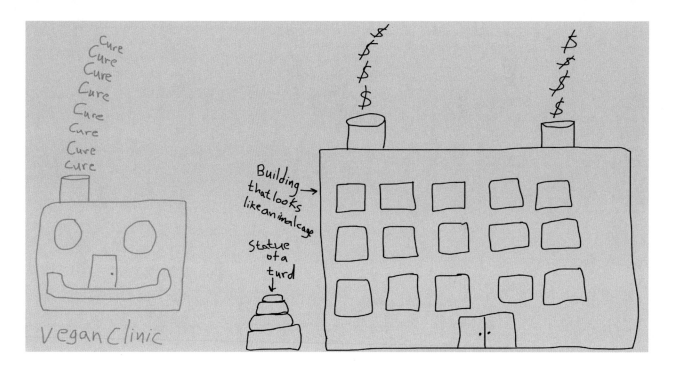

Fig 96: **If you had a little clinic that only taught the vegan, whole food, Spartan diet** and compared it with a big hospital that had all the expensive bells and whistles;

and then compared the patient population, who would have healthier patients?

The big hospital would be better for emergency room care, for high tech stuff like hip replacements, kidney dialysis, kidney transplant;

But the vegan clinic would be better for at least 70% of disease.

"Modern buildings look like animal cages, and they always have a statue of a turn in front." - Tom Wolfe, great American writer.

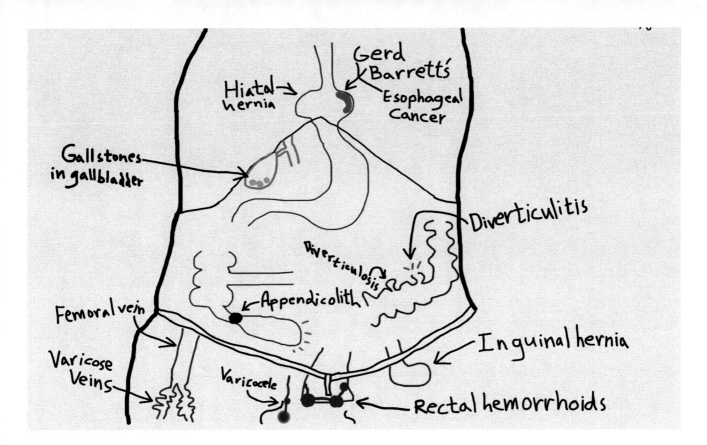

Fig 97: **Abdominal pressure syndrome** as described by Irish missionary physician, Dennis Birkett.

Drawing should also include colon cancer.

Eating adequate amounts of fiber helps to prevent all these diseases.

Fiber comes from plants, because plants stabilize their plasma cell membranes with fiber.

Plant foods do not have any cholesterol.

Animal cells stabilize their plasma cell membranes with cholesterol.

That's why animal foods all have cholesterol.

When you eat plant foods, you get the good stuff, and avoid the bad stuff.

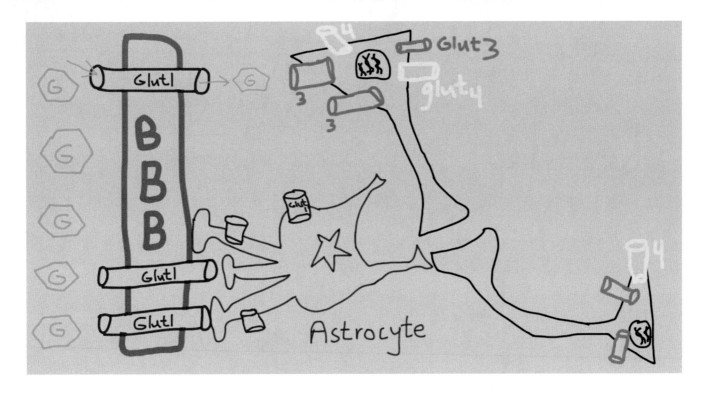

Fig 98: **Brain neurons = brain cells have glucose type 4 transporters (Glut 4).**

Glut 4 transporters are insulin dependent.

Insulin resistance makes glucose less able to enter brain cells.

Less glucose entry can cause dysfunction of these neurons.

This is one of the reasons why diabetes can make you stupid.

The main cause of insulin resistance is high fat diets, especially saturated fat.

Meat and dairy are full of saturated fat.

This is another reason why low fat, whole food, 100% plant based is best diet.

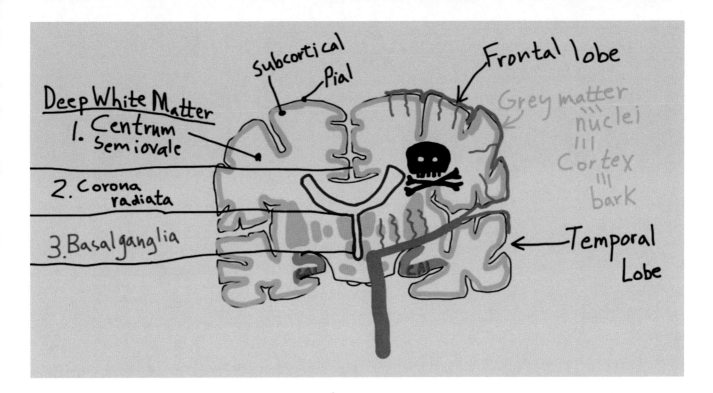

Fig 99: **Excess dietary salt, fat, stress, caffeine, and sleep deprivation cause hypertension.**
Hypertension is the #1 risk factor for atherosclerosis and stroke.

Strokes can make you stupid.

Small strokes are very, very common. I see them every day, all day long.

Overtreatment of hypertension can lead to decreased blood flow to brain; and this can cause cognitive decline.

That's from the Jack de la Torre theory of cerebral hypoperfusion as a very common cause of cognitive decline.

What's the point.

Optimal diet, exercise, sleep, stress management leads to optimal blood pressure & optimal cognitive function.

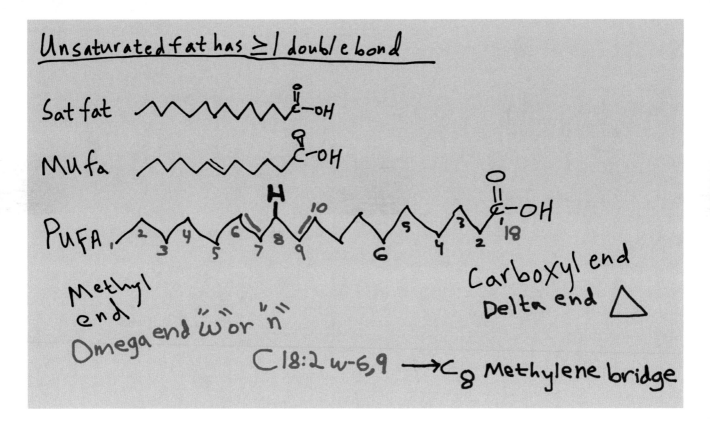

Fig 100: **Fatty acid types.**

Saturated fat is "saturated" with hydrogens. Saturated fat has ZERO double bonds.

MUFA is MonoUnsaturated Fatty Acid.

MUFA has one double bond.

PUFA is PolyUnsaturated Fatty Acid.

PUFA has two or more double bonds.

The two categories of PUFA's are omega 3 and omega 6.

Omega 3 PUFA's have the first double bond at the #3 position (counting from the omega end which is also the methyl end of the fatty acid).

Omega 6 PUFA's have a the first double bond at the omega 6 position.

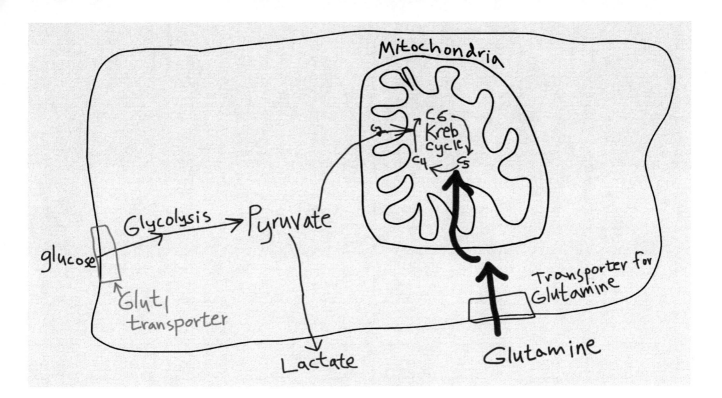

Fig 101: **Glutamine is a common amino acid that can supply the Kreb's cycle** with all the carbon it needs.

What's the point?

Kreb's cycle can run on just glutamine! It doesn't need glucose!

This is one of the many reasons that I think the ketogenic idea is very stupid.

Ketogenic diet tends to be a high animal protein diet; animal protein is a MAJOR tumor promoter.

Ketogenic proponents will say that they want to decrease dietary glucose, to slow down cancer metabolism. But their reasoning is flawed.

Because Kreb's cycle can run on glutamine.

Because animal fat causes insulin resistance!

Because animal protein, fat, iron all cause activation of mTOR!

Because animal fat in the blood causes tissue hypoxia.

Because animal food is typically flavored with salt.

In my opinion, Keto for cancer is stupid!

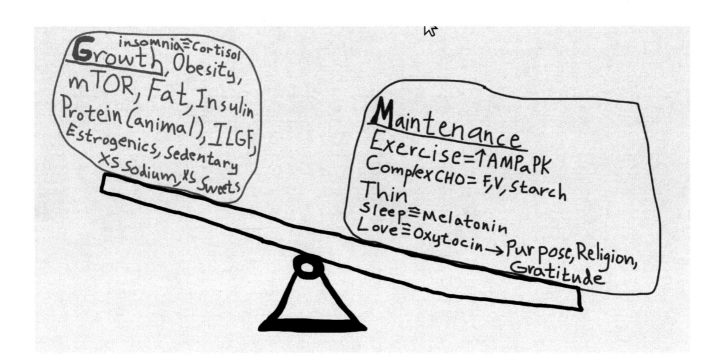

Fig 102: **Goal is to spend as much time as possible in the maintenance phase** = vegan diet, adequate sleep, exercise, adequate sunshine, attitude of gratitude, positive relationships, religion.

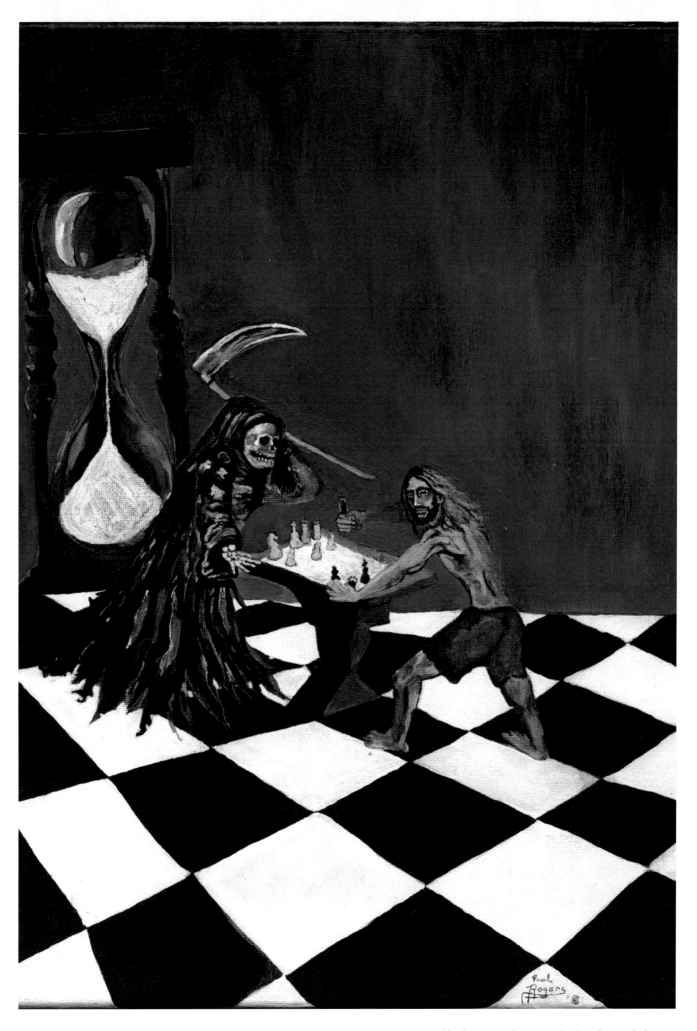

Fig 103: **Playing chess with death** by Paul Rogers, 2023. We are all playing chess with death, and the vegan diet, exercise, sunshine, sleep, love, all help us to live longer.

Most memorable lines in Vegan history = real nutrition history

Carbohydrate

John McDougall → All healthy populations eat a starch based diet. No exceptions.

Dennis Burkitt → High fiber diets protect patients from abdominal pressure syndrome.

Durian Rider → Sugar is the most powerful performance enhancer for your brain, your muscles & your dong!

Peter Rogers → Fruits taste great, but are less filling than starches. [Paraphrase of Mcdougall, but more fun]

Lipid

Caldwell Esselstyn → No oil! Moderation kills. You only see heart disease in the countries that eat a lot of meat and oils. Coronary artery disease is a food borne illness!

Nathan Pritikin → Fat is bad! There is no such thing as a normal occurring diet that's deficient in fat or protein. In studies with controlled diets, people who ate .75% fat did very well.

Roy Swank → Central Norway eats a lot of saturated fat, and they have a lot of MS. Coastal Norway eats much less saturated fat, and they have much less MS. The Chinese diet is mostly rice. It's very low in fat. I don't think there were any MS patients in China.

John McDougall → The fat you eat is the fat you wear!

Jeff Nelson (veg source you tube channel) → The fat in nuts is also bad for blood flow. The benefits of omega three fats are exaggerated.

William Roberts MD → When you feed them a high fat diet, all herbivores get atherosclerosis. Humans are herbivores. Eggs are what you feed an animal to cause atherosclerosis.

Michael Brownlee Phd → Excess dietary fat causes reversal of electron transport in mitochondria. This causes insulin resistance.

Gerald Shulman MD Phd → With nuclear magnetic resonance spectroscopy, we have confirmed that excess fat in skeletal muscle is the main cause of insulin resistance. We call this the "ectopic fat theory" of diabetes.

Peter Rogers → There's no such thing as good fats, except "secret fat." Fiber is good fat. Fiber is safe fat. Unlike other fats, fiber protects you from leaky gut.

Protein

T Colin Campbell → Animal protein is the most powerful tumor promoter.

Walter Kempner → Low protein diet lowers workload of kidneys.

James R Mitchell Phd → the less protein an animal eats, the longer it lives, and that seems to be true for humans too.

Leonard Hayflick → Human somatic cells [most cells in body, not stem cells or germ cells] can only divide about 60 times before they die. That's the Hayflick limit.

Dean Ornish → Plant based diets and stress management help to maintain telomeres, and this slows down aging. [delays arrival at the Hayflick limit].

Peter Rogers → Animal protein has more leucine & methionine than plant protein. Animal foods are also high in fat and iron. All of these things activate mTOR. MTOR causes accelerated rates of cell replication. When you speed up cell replication, you speed up arrival at the Hayflick limit; you speed up aging.

Miscellaneous

Chef AJ → eat your veggies first, if it's in your house, it's in your mouth.

Richard Moore MD Phd → The reason black people have so much HTN is b/c not enough potassium. Populations who eat a plant diet, have same BP in their teens and their 70's.

John Mcdougall → the most common cause of autoimmune disease is leaky gut. The body is always trying to heal.

Dean Ornish → Vegetarian diet and stress management enabled men with biopsy proven low grade prostate cancer to lower their PSA, or at least keep it from increasing.

Ruth Heidrich Phd → The most common cause of disease is ignorance. It only took me two hours to become a vegan, after talking to Dr Mcdougall.

Lorraine Day → You aren't sick, because you have cancer. You have cancer, because you are sick. You need to learn about God's way of healing.

Jack de la Torre Phd → chronic cerebral hypoperfusion [mouse equivalents] is the most common cause of dementia.

Peter Rogers → Neuro vascular uncoupling [mismatch between oxygen delivery & metabolic rate] is most common cause of dementia [de la Torre theory is a subset of this].

Peter Rogers → Healthiest way to live is like Adam & Eve, but with indoor heating and plumbing. The average person is happy that they are not as fat as their cousin, but those are low standards; better to try to be as healthy as you can be; Then you'll be as healthy as you can be.

Peter Rogers → Ischemic spine is the most common cause of back pain [F- & GP make it worse b/c damage collagen].

Michael Greger MD → There's only two categories of nutrition doctors: vegans and those who haven't read the literature yet.

Chapter 5

Text information on cancer

Cancer

What are the three phases of cancer?

#1. **Initiation** = DNA damage = **mutation** = caused by a carcinogen = turns off cell growth regulation.

Some cancer is thought caused by random mutation, otherwise known as bad luck; but just because a cancer is present, that doesn't mean it will grow.

The mutation can be activation of an "oncogene," which means a gene capable of causing cancer;

or a mutation that turns off a "tumor suppressor gene," which means a gene that normally suppresses cancer.

Initiation is emphasized by the **"mutation theory of cancer."**

DNA gets damaged all the time, and the cell is usually good at repairing it.

Genetic vulnerabilities are associated with less ability to repair DNA, and these are emphasized with **"genetic, or family history, theories of cancer."**

#2. **Promotion** = something causes abnormal growth of a cancer cell.

Promotion is emphasized by **"metabolic theory of cancer."**

In reality, cancer causation and growth is a **combination of 1, genetic vulnerabilities, 2. carcinogens inducing mutation, and 3. metabolism.**

#3. **Metastasis** = distant spread of tumor.

Brain and lung metastases often cause death.

People usually don't die from the original primary tumor; they usually die from the metastases.

Women do not die from the tumor in their breast; They die from metastasis.

What are the three main pathways to cancer?

Genetic, mutation, and metabolic. Genetic causes are rare.

Cancer causation is usually a combination of mutation, and abnormal metabolism.

Why do some cells become cancerous?

A normal cell can become "cancerous" when its **"growth control" DNA** is damaged and not repaired.

Cancer growth is suppressed by **tumor suppressor genes,** which include genes **for DNA repair.**

Cancer cells tend to undergo **"aerobic-anaerobic" glycolysis** = burning glucose for energy without using the mitochondria.

The mitochondrial electron transport system is **oxygen** dependent for energy production.

What is the Waarburg effect?

Cancer cells running on glycolysis burn through a lot of glucose, and this is called the Waarburg effect.

"The prime cause of cancer is the replacement of normal oxygen respiration in cells by fermentation [anaerobic glycolysis]."

- Otto Waarburg, Nobel prize winner 1931.

What Otto is saying is that healthy cells **fully** metabolize glucose in healthy mitochondria by transferring electrons to **oxygen**;

Cancer cells only **partially** metabolize glucose;

because cancer cells have **damaged mitochondria**.

Clinical oncologists, surgical oncologists, and radiation therapists are experts on the mutation component of cancer.
This guides choice of chemotherapy, surgery, and radiation therapy.

To also help yourself, you should learn about the benefits of:

- Stress reduction.
- Sleep optimization.
- Simplifying your life so you have time for exercise and sleep.
- Eating low fat vegan to improve the metabolic component of cancer.

You choose what you eat, and that might have a big effect on your cancer rate of growth, according to the research of Ornish, Campbell, Heidrich, McDougall, Pedersen, and others.

What is cancer milieu?

Milieu is the local environment of cancer cells.

Cancer milieu has what key characteristics?

Otto Waarburg noted that different types of cancer tend to produce increased **lactic acid**.

The cancer cells secrete lactic acid into the extracellular matrix.

The immune system normally can remove cancer cells.

Lactic acid **IMPAIRS THE IMMUNE SYSTEM** by blocking activation of CD8+ T and NK cells.

Running on glycolysis enables cancer cells to keep growing in low oxygen conditions.

Cancer cell ability to grow in low oxygen conditions enables cancer cells to **out proliferate the surrounding cells**.

This glycolysis dependent behavior led to the recognition that cancer cells tend to have **MITOCHONDRIAL DYSFUNCTION.**

Cancer cell replication and growth is **"promoted"** by ongoing exposure to conditions that favor cancer growth.
Cancer cells tend to develop a localized **hypoxic, acidotic milieu.**

Hypoxic, acidotic milieu.

Hypoxic, acidotic milieu.

Normal cells do not function well in a hypoxic, acidotic milieu.

A hypoxic, acidotic milieu enables cancer cells to outgrow neighboring cells.

What are tumor promoters?

Things that favor cancer growth.

The common tumor promoters are:

- **Alcohol,**
- **Tobacco,**
- **Animal protein,**
- **Animal fat,**
- **Oils,**
- **Estrogenics**

What's the significance of tumor promoters?

Everyone has been exposed to carcinogens. Everyone has some DNA mutations.

Almost all of these will be of no significance.

You certainly should avoid carcinogens when you can, but it is more important to **FOCUS ON AVOIDING TUMOR PROMOTERS.**

It usually takes multiple decades for a cancer to become clinically relevant.

Our bodies are GREAT at repairing damaged DNA.

The smart move is to avoid tumor promoters so that a mutant cell never gets activated to become a clinically relevant cancer.

What is an easy way to remember the common tumor promoters?

Anything that's bad for your arteries probably increases the risk of cancer.

What's good for the heart is good for the brain, and helps prevent cancer.

What can a person do to try to decrease the risk of cancer growth?

You want to promote a well oxygenated, normal pH milieu!

Vegan diet prevents rouleaux, and hypertension, and atherosclerosis, and therefore tends to increase **oxygen** delivery to tissues.

Vegan diet is **alkaline** compared to meat diet. Just eat vegan foods. Do not go doing other crazy stuff about alkalinity. Your blood has to maintain a pH of around 7.4.

The key point is the **LOCAL** milieu of the cancer.

What about reducing animal protein?

Vegan diet is low in the essential amino acids called leucine and methionine.

Cancer needs lots of leucine and methionine for making proteins, and replicating DNA.

Cancer needs lots of nitrogen for making proteins and replicating DNA.

T Colin Campbell's research showed that when animal protein gets over 10% of calories, there is a big increase in cancer risk.

Cancer especially ramps up metabolism of glutamine which is a "conditionally" essential amino acid.

Plant diets help to deprive cancer of the leucine and methionine that cancer wants. Vegan diet reduces the risk of getting cancer.

The average person "wants" to eat more animal protein. A well informed person fears animal protein, and avoids it.

What about prostate cancer?

Prostate cancer is hormonal, similar to breast cancer; increased risk with estrogenic chemicals.

It ain't the young guys with high testosterone who get prostate cancer. It's the old guys with low testosterone who get prostate cancer.

Check out the research of Dr. Ornish on diet and PSA.

What causes mitochondrial dysfunction?

- **Hypoxia**.

    - Hypoxia causes dysfunction because oxygen is needed to serve as the ultimate electron acceptor in electron transport.
    - Otto Waarburg showed in the 1920's that when cells are hypoxic, they sometimes become cancerous.

- **Saturated fat.**

    - Saturated fat, beta-oxidation yields the maximum number of $FADH_2$ electron carriers, and this tends to overwhelm electron transport between coenzyme Q and complex 3.
    - Saturated fat causes reversal of electron transport, and increased production of ROS.

- **Intracellular hyperglycemia.**

    - Some cells are not glut 4 (insulin dependent glucose type 4 transporter) dependent.
    - These cells take up glucose continuously, and in the presence of hyperglycemia, can be flooded by glucose.
    - This INTRAcellular HYPERglycemia can also overwhelm electron transport, and lead to it's reversal.
    - INTRAcellular HYPERglycemia is typically caused by poorly controlled, insulin dependent diabetes.

- **PUFA's (PolyUnsaturated Fatty Acids)**

    - PUFA's are vulnerable to lipid peroxidation, especially in the setting of free-unliganded iron.
    - Lipid peroxidation can set off a chain reaction — like dominos — in mitochondrial membranes.
    - Mitochondrial membranes contain a lot of PUFA's.

- **Mitochondrial toxins,** like some pesticides. Pesticides tend to bioaccumulate in nonorganic meat.

In addition to hypoxia, saturated fat, intracellular hyperglycemia, and free iron, what else can generate a lot of ROS?

The enzyme, NADPH oxidase which is sometimes abbreviated Nox.

Nox can be "overactivated" by AGE's. AGE's are Advanced Glycation Endproducts.

Hyperglycemia (excess glucose in the blood caused by diabetes) can glycate proteins to form AGE's.

Hemoglobin A1-C is a blood test that indicates glycation.

AGE's can bind Receptors for AGE's that are called R-AGE receptors.

Binding of AGE's to R-AGE receptors causes activation of NADPH Oxidase, and generation of ROS, like superoxide anions.

What stimulates a cell to grow, and possibly proliferate?

- Insulin is anabolic.

- ILGF (Insulin Like Growth Factor) is anabolic.

- Estrogen stimulates cell proliferation in the breast, endometrium, and prostate.

- Leucine is a branched chain, amino acid that stimulates mTOR. MTOR is a nutrient sensing system, and a growth regulator.

- When mTOR senses that nutrients are widely available, it "tells" the cells to grow.

- MTOR overactivation is thought to contribute to growth in the majority of cancers.

- Methionine is an essential amino acid for cancer growth. Meat has much more methionine, than do plant foods.

What causes DNA mutations?

Carcinogen chemicals, tobacco smoke, alcohol, hypoxia, insulin resistance. Deficiencies of folate and vitamin B12.

Anything that increases oxidative stress, like PUFA's, and unliganded iron, can increase mutations. Oxidative stress means increased reactive oxygen species (ROS). ROS can cause mutations.

What is a proto-oncogene?

A proto-oncogene is a gene, that if mutated could cause cancer.

What is an oncogene?

An oncogene is a gene that is contributing to the cause of cancer.

What is p53?
P53 is a tumor suppressor gene because it helps for DNA repair.

- p53 is sometimes called "the guardian of the genome."
- p53 protein helps recognize double stranded DNA breaks.
- p53 then activates a pathway to repair the DNA.
- If the DNA cannot be repaired, then p53 signals for the cell go into apoptosis.
- Mutations in p53 cause increased risk of cancer.
- P53 mutation is the most common mutation in cancers.
- Benzpyrene, a carcinogen in cigarettes, binds the p53 gene, leading to cancer.

Things that decrease risk of cancer:

Vegan diet.

- No animal protein.

  - That's right! **ZERO** animal protein!

- Fish is not okay.

  - It's all animal muscle.
  - Animal muscle means animal protein, and saturated fat.
  - All animal muscle should be avoided.
  - Even if it's grass fed, it's still got animal protein and saturated fat.

- Even a small amount of animal protein can cause a big increase in risk of cancer.

- The graph of cancer frequency vs meat consumption is linear, about a 45 degree line, with about 1:1 correlation between meat intake, and cancer rate, and it goes through zero;

- there is no safe amount of meat, not associated with an increase risk of cancer.

- **Meat is unsafe "at any speed."**

- Even animal protein intakes as low as 3% of calories appear to be associated with increased risk of cancer.

- Therefore, you want ZERO, none, nada, not one bite, not one nanometer!

- Plant foods are super low in saturated fat.

- Plant foods have lots of **ANTIOXIDANTS** like vitamin C.

- Green vegetables like salad and broccoli, often increase **NITRIC OXIDE** and blood flow.

- Greens are **ALKALINE**, and thus help prevent acidosis.

AVOID ANIMAL PROTEIN.

- Animal protein causes increased blood cholesterol, and atherosclerosis. (That's not a misprint. Animal PROTEIN does cause increased cholesterol).
- Animal protein is a tumor promoter.

- Animal protein increases ILGF.
- Leucine is more common in animal protein.

  - Leucine activates mTOR, a nutrient sensing, growth regulator.

  - When large amounts of leucine are present, mTOR "senses" nutrients are widely available, and might increase cell growth and proliferation.

- Methionine is more common in animal protein.
  - Cancer cells want more methionine.

AVOID ANIMAL FAT.

- Animal fat means saturated fat.

- Animal fat increase is associated with increased risk of cancer.

- Populations that do not eat meat or oils, have an amazingly low incidence of breast cancer.

- The more animal fat a person eats, the higher their risk of cancer.

- In countries where people eat a lot of animal fat, there is a lot of colon cancer, breast cancer, and prostate cancer.

- Saturated fat causes RBC rouleaux, and tissue hypoxia.

- Saturated fat tends to cause mitochondrial dysfunction.

- Animal fat causes increased cholesterol level.

- Increased cholesterol is associated with increased risk of atherosclerosis and cancer.

- The chemical formula for cholesterol is $C_{27}H_{46}O$.

- High cholesterol can lead to increased production of a cholesterol metabolite called, **27-hydroxy-cholesterol.**

- Some cancers, like tamoxifen resistant breast cancer, sometimes feed on 27-hydroxy-cholesterol.

- The enzyme Cyp27-A1 converts cholesterol into 27-hydroxy cholesterol.

- 27 hydroxy-cholesterol can have an estrogenic, tumor promoting effect on breast cancer cells.

- Some speculate that 27 hydroxy-cholesterol can contribute to reactivation of breast cancer in some patients, such as those that are resistant to tamoxifen.

- 27-hydroxy-cholesterol appears to be a tumor promoter that might increase the risk of breast cancer metastases.

- The ideal cholesterol is TOTAL cholesterol always below 150.

- Note: this is **TOTAL** cholesterol below 150.

- Total cholesterol below 150 is the key therapeutic goal for preventing atherosclerosis, (which is another way of saying, increasing tissue oxygenation).

- If your total cholesterol is below 150, your LDL will be okay. However, if you want a number goal for LDL, then try to get it down to 60 mg/dl.

Eat starch to:

- Provide fiber, and prevent leaky gut; thus reduce inflammation.
- Provide fiber and promote gut flora that increases estrogen removal from the body by defecation.

Eat fruits and vegetables:

- High in antioxidants, like vitamin C, which protect DNA, and mitochondria.
- Lower blood viscosity, which improves blood flow, which prevents hypoxia.
- Alkaline to possibly decrease cancer related acidotic milieu.
- Low in methionine and leucine.
- Cruciferous vegetables are thought especially protective, like broccoli, and brussel sprouts.

Exercise.

- Exercise dramatically decreases risk of breast cancer; and the more the exercise, the more the risk reduction.
- 11 minutes of walking reduces risk by 20%. 4 hrs/week reduces risk by 40%. 5 or more hours per week reduces risk by about 60%.
- Kind of reminds you of triathletes like Ruth Heidrich.
- Everybody knows that walking contracts leg muscles which squeeze the veins, and this helps return blood to the heart.
- Everybody knows that the leg veins have valves to facilitate unidirectional blood flow.
- But did you know that there's another system of "vessels with valves" in your legs; and throughout your body?

It's called the LYMPHATIC SYSTEM!!!

When you walk, you get your lymph to flow. When your lymph flows, your WBC's travel around the body to search for cancer cells, and remove them.

What are the other benefits of exercise?

- Walking helps your WBC's to do their job of protecting you.

    - Exercise increases nitric oxide vasodilator to open up arteries.

    - Exercise improves tissue perfusion.

    - Exercise improves physical appearance.

    - Exercise improves self esteem.

    - Exercise lowers stress levels.

Sleep at night.

At least one good social relationship.

- *Social support increases survival with breast cancer.*

Helping at least one other person on a routine basis.

    - Improves self esteem.

- Lowers stress levels.

- When you help others, you help yourself.

- A mood booster because of reward neurotransmitters that approve of you doing things that will help you to maintain acceptance by the social group.

Love

- To be loved makes a person feel safe which lowers their stress levels.

- To love someone and try to help them gives a person a sense of purpose.

  - A sense of purpose lowers stress levels.

A purpose in life

- Energizes a person.

- Improves self esteem.

- Increased happiness.

Avoid things that increase cancer risk.

Carcinogens include:
- Benzopyrene in cigarette smoke.
- Heterocyclic amines in meat.
- Alcohol,
- Asbestos.
- Aflatoxin,
- Arsenic,
- Benzene,
- Dioxin.

Genetic vulnerabilities to cancer.

- BRCA1 and BRCA2 genes are involved in DNA repair.
- Women with defects in either the BRCA1 or BRCA2 genes have increased risk of breast cancer.

EDC's

EDC's increase risk of breast cancer, and that is covered in other chapters of this book.

Be careful what you put in your mouth; alcohol, mouthwash, toothpaste, tobacco can all be carcinogenic and/or estrogenic.

SEDENTARY

ALUMINUM

Armpit and breast lymphatics are connected.

Breast cancer (BC) is most common in the upper outer quadrant (UOQ).

UOQ BC has increased percentage wise in past century.

Theory is that armpit aluminum deodorant increases BC risk.

Aluminum is a "metalloestrogen" that can stimulate growth of BC.

BC risk is increased if a woman shaves first, before applying aluminum, because nicks in skin can increase absorption.

Humans are not dogs.

We don't greet each other by sniffing butts or armpits.

You don't need to wear deodorant!

EDC's (Estrogen Disrupting Chemicals) from other skin care products like sunscreen, and paraben preservatives, can increase risk of cancer.

ALCOHOL

Beverage alcohol is ethanol, C-C-OH. Ethanol is converted in liver to acetaldehyde, C-CH=O.

Acetaldehyde is thought to be carcinogenic and increase BC risk.
Alcohol decreases immune function. Alcohol can lead to decreased thiamine, with resultant decreased cognitive function.

Alcohol can decrease folate, which can lead to impaired DNA synthesis, which leads to uracils being inserted into DNA, instead of Thymines, with resultant increased mutations.

Liver conversion of ethanol to acetaldehyde and acetate, C-C=O & O- generates NADPH which signals to store fats (instead of burn them) leading to fatty liver.

Alcohol effect on fat metabolism apparently is the reason that alcohol "stiffens" red blood cell (RBC) cell membranes.

Stiff RBC's means less flexible RBC's.

Less flexible RBC's means increased blood viscosity.

Increased blood viscosity means high blood pressure.

High blood pressure causes atherosclerosis.

Atherosclerosis causes tissue hypoxia.

Tissue hypoxia favors cancer cells.

Alcohol is a tumor promoter.

Increased alcohol causes increased risk of head and neck cancers.

Head and neck cancer cancers are bad cancers.

Head and neck cancer surgery routinely removes the tongue and the larynx (voicebox).

Alcohol also increases risk of esophageal cancer.

Esophageal cancer is a bad cancer.

The last thing in the world that I would want to do, is pour a tumor promoter, over my tongue, and larynx, and esophagus.

I do not drink alcohol.

Not one drop.

Breast cancer risk factors:

95% of breast cancer patients are over 40 years old when diagnosed. The median age of breast cancer diagnosis is 62 years old. Why is it that older women with "low" estrogen production, get breast cancer, instead of older women with "high" estrogen production?

Maybe because older women are fatter, and the fat tissue has the enzyme "aromatase," to make estrogen. Maybe it's because of the increased accumulation of estrogenic chemicals, and because their immune systems are weaker, and they have more atherosclerosis.

Anything that increases estrogen (unopposed).

- Obesity is the most probably the most important controllable risk factor.
- Early menarche.
- Late menopause.
- Nulliparity.
- Late age of childbearing.
- No breast feeding.
- Long term OCP's (oral contraceptive pills).
- Long term HRT (hormone replacement therapy).
- Estrogenic chemicals in deodorants, and other cosmetic products.
- Estrogenic chemicals in laundry detergents.
- Chemicals in processed food and meat like pesticides, herbicides, and food dyes as some of these are estrogenic.
- Drinking water that contains high levels of estrogenic chemicals.

Other general risk factors for cancer:

- High animal protein diet.
- High animal fat diet.
- Alcohol.
- Tobacco.
- Obesity.
- Diabetes.
- Sedentary.
- Silicone gel breast implants, especially if wrapped in polyurethane foam.
- Dark hair dyes with prolonged use.
- Electric blankets.
- Cleaning chemicals.
- Live near gas station or refinery.
- Lack of sleep.
- BRCA is a tumor suppressor gene that when mutated causes increased risk of breast cancer. 90-95% of breast cancer is not genetic. 87% of breast cancer patients do not have any first degree relatives with breast cancer. If an identical twin has breast cancer, her twin only has a 20% increase in risk of breast cancer; same as if her nontwin sister had breast cancer.

Read about cancer

- Read the work of T. Colin Campbell PhD, Kristi Funk MD (she wrong about soy), Dean Ornish MD (on prostate cancer), Dr. John Kelly, Ruth Heidrich PhD, Lorraine Day MD, and others.

- Consider join a support group so can talk to someone about life with cancer.

What is the connection between excess estrogen and cancer?

Elevated estrogen increases risk of breast cancer, endometrial cancer, and prostate cancer.

Persons who eat a lot of animal fat, tend to become fat themselves, which increases estrogen levels.

Eating **MEAT INCREASES ESTROGEN LEVELS** because meat causes a change in gut bacteria.

Normally, estrogen is conjugated in the liver, and then excreted in the stool.

Meat induced gut bacteria **cause DECONJUGATION of estrogen** so that it is reabsorbed back into the body.

This is called the enterohepatic circulation.

Meat related RE-absorption of estrogen causes increased blood levels of estrogen.

Meat eaters have higher blood levels of estrogen.

Plant eaters poop out their excess estrogen.

Fiber essentially PULLS ESTROGEN OUT OF YOUR BODY.

Yea!

Female meat eaters have increased breast carcinoma, and uterine fibroids.

Female vegetarians are less likely to get breast cancer.

Populations that eat a low fat vegan diet, have low rates of breast and prostate cancer.

Populations that eat moderate to high amounts of meat have high rates of breast and prostate cancer.

Does that mean it's okay to eat small amounts of meat?

No!

As cancer grows, it acquires more mutations, and becomes more aggressive, more malignant.

I've read about a lot of cancer patients who were in remission, and then they went back to old habits of eating meat, and oils, and salt, and their cancer came back, and killed them.

Some cancers have **OVEREXPRESSION OF RECEPTORS** for growth factors which can lead to an amplified growth response.

Do not take a chance. My advice is do not take one bite of meat ever again in your life. And no oils.

My guess is that cancer cells can become **SENSITIZED** to growth factors, such that even small amounts of meat related tumor promoters might have a big effect.

There are times in life when you must move on to better things, and don't look back.

Lot's wife looked back, and she was turned into a pillar of salt.

Orpheus looked back, and Eurydice was dragged back into Hell.

How come older woman get more breast cancer even though they are postmenopausal with decreasing endogenous estrogen levels?

Older persons have weaker immune systems.

Older persons have accumulated lots of estrogenic chemicals from aluminum deodorant, skin moisturizers-sunscreen-colognes-perfumes, laundry detergent, and eating meat.

From what I've seen, women love to rub cosmetic "crap" on themselves. My mom used to do that, and she died of cancer.

My wife has about 55 cosmetic products that she rubs on herself. I told her that she is a stupid monkey playing with chemicals that she doesn't understand.

Wife: You don't understand. A woman would rub sh_t on her face, if she thought it would make her pretty.

Me: That's a big assumption, to think this stuff is going to make you prettier. These magic creams are not going to help you to lose weight.

Wife: I'm not fat. I'm just chubby. It's okay to be a little chubby.

I have ZERO cosmetic products. I do not use deodorant. I do not use sunscreen. I do not use laundry detergent.

Guess who is aging better. I look about 15 years younger than her. When we got married, she was a superfox, 10/10; now she puts her hopes in wrinkle creams that don't work.

I told her to become a vegan, and she is trying to move in that direction, but she doesn't read books.

I think a person has to read books.

When you read about nutrition, and estrogen, and cancer, it's obvious that the best strategy is to become a low fat, vegan, cosmetic minimalist.

Advanced discussion of Cancer

Monoclonal origin

- Cancer is thought to arise from a single cell of origin.
- Human cells normally work together for the benefit of the entire body.
- Cancer cells have broken out of the normal, altruistic mode, and now are just reproducing in their own "selfish" mode.
- Cell growth = cell gets bigger.
- Cell division = cell replicates.

Contact inhibition = normal cells express cell surface chemicals, that tell other cells adjacent to them, that they should not replicate; to prevent crowding.

- Cancer is human cells behaving badly; like bacteria; out for themselves, instead of for the whole organism.

- **Presumed carcinogens** = tobacco, alcohol, estrogenic chemicals, aluminum, benzene, aflatoxin, tumor viruses (HBV, HCV), oils, meat.

Cancer causation by mutation is called the **"Somatic Mutation Theory" or SMT.**

- SMT says that somatic cells (means non-germ cells) undergo mutations;
    - the mutations enable them to proliferate out of control.
- Most cancers are thought to originally come from one cell; and this is called the "monoclonal origin of a tumor."
    - However, mutations occur within the cells of a malignant tumor.

- Cancers eventually tend to develop a **wide variety of mutations.**
    - The same tumor can have different mutations in different cells, and this is called "**intra-tumoral heterogeneity**."

    - Intra-tumoral heterogeneity can decrease the likelihood of response to monotherapy.

    - Tumoral heterogeneity is a major problem.

    - Tumoral heterogeneity means that CANCER tends to become MORE AGGRESSIVE over time.

    - The bigger the tumor gets, the more mutated it tends to get.

    - Cancer can turn into an uncontrollable monster.

The point is that you want to prevent it if possible, and certainly **do NOT give it any tumor promoters.**

- No meat. Not one bite.
- That means no milk, no cheese, no yogurt, no fish. Not one bite.
- No oils. That includes no olive oil. Not one drop.
- No alcohol. Not one sip.
- No tobacco. Not one puff.
- I've seen tons of people die from cancer.
- The best option is to try to prevent it.
- If you already have it, then optimize your health to perfection, and hopefully you will be able to slow it down.
- Lots of studies show that optimizing health by optimizing nutrition (most important thing), exercise, sunshine, social support, purpose, and avoiding psychological stress, can often lead to a big improvement in outcome.

The rationale goes like this:

Okay, Mr Cancer, you may have made a little spot for yourself inside of me, but I'm gonna make you wish you were somewhere else.

- I will NOT give you any tumor promoters.

- I will alkalinize your milieu with plant foods.

- I will increase oxygen delivery by eating a low fat, low salt plant food diet.

- I will also increase oxygen delivery with exercise.

- I will improve immune function with exercise.

- I will lower cortisol by avoiding unnecessary stress and caffeine.

- I will be nice to people, and maintain my social support, so that I can spend more time in a parasympathetic mood, which improves healing.

- I will avoid milk and other excesses of calcium, and go out in the sun, to get more 1,25-hydroxy vitamin D — the active form.

- I will help at least one other person every day, for their sake, and for mine, because somehow being good to others, energizes our souls to want to live.

"Believe that life is worth living, and your belief will help create the fact."
- William James.

"Does faith spring from miracles, or do miracles spring from faith?"
- Dostoevsky.

My Mom had a 2 year prognosis, but lived 11 years.

She did great with all the social stuff; minister of care, director of an orphanage, tour guide for art museum, tour guide for architecture, tennis player, charming, funny personality.

But she screwed up by continuing to eat meat and oils. At the time, I didn't know enough to advise her.

- Critics of the SMT say that mitochondrial dysfunction — a metabolic problem — is the initiating event — that leads to mutations.
    - In other words, mitochondrial dysfunction leads to increased reactive oxygen species (ROS), and advanced glycation endproducts (AGEs);
    - and the ROS and AGE's then cause the mutations;
    - and that's why the mutation pattern is so variable.

- The Cancer Genome Atlas project (TCGA) showed that cancer mutations are relatively random.

Metabolic theory of cancer (MTC) posits that cancer is mostly driven by metabolic factors.

- Travis Christofferson wrote a book called "**Tripping over the truth**" about metabolic theory.
- Christofferson's book is a great book for pathophysiology — one of the best — but it screws up on diet recommendations.
- I actually do think it's a great book, and that all cancer patients should read it.
- Christofferson's book provides the scientific background to understand cancer in a sophisticated way.
- Christofferson is really good at explaining the historical development of research into cancer related physiology, and genetics, and therapy.
- I was impressed by the entire book except the high fat diet recommendation.
- However, because of the importance of the topic, and the desire to help the cancer patients, I must correct the dietary recommendations of Seyfried and Christofferson.

Waarburg, Pederson, Hee Ko, Seyfried, McDougall and Campbell are some of the most famous researchers to promote the metabolic theory of cancer.

Otto Waarburg, biochemist noticed that different types of cancer all tended to produce lactic acid **(Waarburg effect).**

- Otto believed that cancer was primarily a **metabolic disease;**
- Otto believed that **hypoxia** causes **mitochondrial dysfunction.**

- Others, who agree with Waarburg, believe that mitochondrial dysfunction then leads to DNA **mutations**.
- Tissue hypoxia as could be caused by rouleaux of RBC's can lead to mitochondrial dysfunction.
- Saturated fat related excess intramyocellular lipid can lead to excess beta oxidation and excess NADH and FADH2 electron carriers going to electron transport.
- The excess electrons can lead to an excess voltage gradient across the inner mitochondrial membrane.
- The excess voltage gradient can lead to electon transport dysfunction which means mitochondrial dysfunction.
- Damaged mitochondria can die.
- Cancer cells have a diminished number of mitochondria.
- The remaining mitochondria are often abnormally small, or deformed in shape.

Cells with depleted mitochondria often die by necrosis or apoptosis.

The cancer cell is the rare cell that was hypoxic, but instead of dying by apoptosis, it mutated, and shifted to anaerobic metabolism.

- In the process of becoming anaerobic, it **dedifferentiated**.
- To dedifferentiate means to stop caring about the cells around itself; to stop trying to be part of an organ like the breast, or the prostate, or the colon; **to only care about itself**;
- to only care about surviving itself, and to hell with it's old duties.
- The cancer cell has **REVERSE EVOLVED** to become like an anaerobic bacteria that just wants to grow as fast as it can,
- In order to grow it wants methionine, and leucine.

Cancer cells often induce or acquire certain metabolic patterns.

- **The mutation to increase hexokinase 2, also prevents apoptosis.**

Cancer types

- Cancer of an epithelial cell is called a **carcinoma**.
  - Most cancers are carcinomas, about 80%.
  - Epithelial cells are thought vulnerable to cancer, because they tend to have intrinsically high rates of cell replication.
- Cancer of lymphocytes is called a **lymphoma**.
- Cancer of connective tissues are called **sarcomas**, and are rare.
- Cancers of blood cells include **leukemias** and **myelomas**.
- Cancers of pigment cells are called **melanomas**.

*"The human body has an amazing capacity **to repair damaged DNA**. If this ability is supported through proper nutrition, most if not all of the damage can be undone long before cancer is initiated…*

Probably 97 to 98% of all cancers are related to diet and lifestyle, and not to genes...

None of the accepted "causes" of cancer in the absence of high animal protein diet mattered that much. Not genetics, not chemical carcinogens, not viruses." - TC Campbell from "Whole, rethinking science of nutrition."

Cancer Metabolism

- Accumulation of **lactic acid** suggests the cancer cells are generating energy from glycolysis in cytoplasm, rather than oxidative phosphorylation in mitochondria.

- **Anaerobic metabolism** enables a cancer cell to grow farther from capillaries;
    - Allows cancer cells to pump lactate into the extracellular space
    - causing acidosis
    - that can get adjacent cells to induce **ANGIOGENESIS**.

- Lactate accumulation can cause increased hypoxia inducible factor (HIF), which leads to increased VEGF for angiogenesis.

- Glycolysis provides substrates for cell replication.

- Anaerobic metabolism enables cell to survive even with mitochondrial dysfunction.

- Lactate can be sent to liver for conversion into glucose via gluconeogenesis.

- **One way to prevent angiogenesis is to PREVENT HYPOXIA.**

- **To prevent hypoxia you need to improve blood flow!!!**

- **To improve blood flow, you need to eat low fat, low salt, whole food, plant based diet.**

- *"**High fat meal decreases PO2 by 20%**… Waarburg said that he could turn normal cells in tissue culture into cancer cells by depriving them of oxygen."*   - John McDougall MD.

- **Some say glycolysis excess in cancer cells is mainly because the cell wants to use glycolytic intermediates for synthesis;**
- because dividing cells need more synthesis to get ready for cell duplication.

- **This is the main theory mentioned in current pathology textbooks.**

- Others say that the reason the cell relies on glycolysis, is because there is mitochondrial dysfunction.

    - Proponents of this theory believe, that if mitochondrial function could be improved,

    - then the patient would likely improve.

- F-DG PET scan is based on the Waarburg effect.
    - Cancer cells can take up 100x as much glucose as normal cells. This can lead to cachexia.
    - Waarburg effect helps cancer cells to grow in hypoxic conditions.

On the one hand, I admire Seyfried and Christofferson for improving knowledge of the metabolic theory of cancer.

On the other hand, I think they are wrong about recommending a high fat diet, because both saturated fat, and PUFA's are harmful to mitochondria.

Both saturated fat and PUFA's cause atherosclerosis, and atherosclerosis leads to hypoxia, and hypoxia favors cancer.

High fat diet means high meat diet, and high meat means high leucine, and methionine. Leucine and methionine appear to promote cancer growth.

High meat diet means increased metabolic acidosis, and acidosis favors cancer.

Seyfried and Christofferson have more direct experience in cancer research than I do, and can say that I'm just a blowhard who does not do research, and does not take care of cancer patients.

Even though that's true, I know I'm right.

Go ahead.

Read about it yourself.

- The **metabolic theory of cancer and the vegan diet** are not very popular because nobody makes money off them, and because most people are too ignorant to ever try to understand them.

- It would be easier to teach my dog sign language, than to get the average American to eat a vegan diet.

Metastasis

- **Metastases** = distant spread of cancer.
- Metastasis is the main reason that people die from cancer.
- Cancer kills by metastasis.

Metastasis is a multistep process that includes:

- Enlargement of the tumor size, beyond 2 mm, requires angiogenesis.
- Hypoxia of a tumor leads to increased HIF (Hypoxia Inducible Factor). Vitamin C helps prevent HIF activation.
- Increased HIF leads to increased VEGF (Vascular Endothelial Growth Factor).
- Metastatic spread requires that the tumor detaches from adjacent tumor cells.
- The cancer cell must then invade its own epithelial basement membrane.
- The cancer cell must then lyse its way through the adjacent extracellular matrix (ECM) connective tissue.
- Vitamin C helps make strong collagen, which might make it harder for cancer cells to lyse their way through ECM.

- Once the cancer cell has travelled through the ECM, it has to dig its way through the endothelial, basement membrane, tight junctions.

- Then the cancer cell has to INTRAvasate itself into a vein or lymphatic vessel.

- The cancer cell interacts with the immune system in the blood, and the lymphatics, and must survive this.

- The cancer cell is carried to its metastatic destination which is most often the lung, but can be anywhere including the liver, bones, or brain.

- Tumor must now repeat the above process in reverse = EXTRAVAsate into ECM.

    - Travel through ECM.
    - Grow in new location.
    - Induce angiogenesis.

- These are a lot of steps. That's why it usually takes decades for cancer to grow and metastasize.

- That's why a person should try to "slow down" the cancer by optimizing their health.

- **Standard treatments for cancer**

  - Surgery for focal tumors.
  - Radiation for nonresectable tumors.
  - Chemotherapy for treatment of primary tumors, micrometastases, and macrometastases.

Cancer cell properties:

- Mutations are common like in P53 gene.

- Cell might have problem with DNA repair. Vitamin C helps maintain DNA.

- **Cell might be overstimulated by growth factors like:**

  - ILGF 1 = increased by animal protein.
  - Insulin = increased by fat = meat and oils.
  - Estrogen = increased by meat.
  - Estrogenic chemicals = EDC's
- Mitochondrial dysfunction.
- Dependence on amino acids like those more common in meat.
- Grows in a hypoxic, acidotic milieu.

Why is the milieu acidic?

- Because cancer cells primarily produce energy from glycolysis.
- Glycolysis generates NADH. But the NADH has "nowhere to go." The NADH cannot send its electrons to electron transport, because mitochondria are dysfunctional.
- Therefore, the cell needs to find a new way to regenerate NAD+, so it can keep running glycolysis.
- Glycolysis requires NAD+ to run.
- The cancer cell solves the problem by converting pyruvate to **lactate**.
- During the conversion of pyruvate to lactate, NAD+ is regenerated.
- The lactate is then secreted into the extracellular matrix to create an acidotic milieu.
- The acidotic milieu favors growth of the cancer cell relative to other cells.
- The acidotic milieu also deactivates immune system cells — CD8 T cells and NK cells — which protects the cancer cells from the immune system.
- To some extent, cancer can be thought of as **reverse embryology** and **reverse evolution**.
- Cancer cells are "immortal" and can keep dividing; cancer cells have telomerase, and do not have a **Hayflick limit**.
- Cancer cells have uncontrolled proliferation, behaving like bacteria.
- Normal cells exposed to hypoxia have a tendency to die by necrosis or apoptosis.
- Cancer cells are unique in their overproduction of **hexokinase 2**;

  - Hexokinase 2 binds to mitochondria.
  - Hexokinase 2 blocks mitochondrial induced apoptosis.
  - Hexokinase 2 sucks up glucose like a vacuum cleaner.
  - Cancer cells burn through tons of glucose, and that's why cancer cells are hot on FDG PET.
  - Remember, that the glucose levels in diabetes are high because the fat has messed up glucose metabolism, NOT because the patient eats glucose.

- Cancer cells have a massive uptake of glucose. Cancer cells use glucose for energy, and for synthesis.

- When glucose enters the cell, it is phosphorylated to become glucose 6-phosphate. Glucose 6-phosphate is of course the beginning of glycolysis.

- Glucose 6-phosphate can be diverted into the **pentose phosphate pathway (PPP)**.

- **PPP is also called Hexose MonoPhosphate (HMP) shunt.**

- PPP is used to make ribose for DNA and RNA synthesis.

- To replicate itself, a cell must make a copy of it's DNA; all **3.2 billion base pairs**. That's a lot of **ribose**.

    - That requires a lot of nitrogen for nucleotide bases, the purines and pyrimidines.
    - That requires a lot of PROTEIN intake.
    - That requires a lot of methionine, and leucine.

Phospholipid synthesis

- For replication, cancer cells also have to make a lot of phospholipids for **plasma cell membranes**, and membranes of organelles.
- Glycolysis provides dihyroxyacetone phosphate (**DHAP**) to serve as the carbon skeleton backbone for phospholipids.

- Cell has to replicate its contents:

    - Protein 55%
    - Nucleic acids 25%
    - Lipids 15%
    - CHO 5%

HYPOXIA

- Rouleaux causes mild hypoxia.

- Rouleaux reduces PO2 by 20%.

- Most people have a large amount of reserve, so a 20% drop in PO2 is not noticed by them.

- But, in elderly patients with comorbidities, 20% drop in PO2 is a big deal.

- Hypoxia causes upregulation of **Hypoxia Inducible Factor (HIF).**

    - HIF is a transcription factor.

- **HIF-1** activates genes for **INCREASED SYNTHESIS OF GLUT 1 & 3 TRANSPORTERS** to increase the basal rate of glucose uptake by cancer cells.

- Increased glut 1 & 3 transporters enables the cancer cell to survive better than "normal cells," in a hypoxic milieu.

- HIF-1 activates production of **INCREASED ENZYMES FOR GLYCOLYSIS**, including hexokinase, phosphofructokinase (PFK), and aldolase.

    - This increases glycolysis in the cell.
    - Cancer runs on **glycolysis**.
- HIF also increases production of **Pyruvate DeHydrogenase Kinase (PDHK-1).**

- PDHK-1 inhibits Pyruvate DeHydrogenase (PDH).

    - Thus, pdhK blocks the conversion of pyruvate by PDH into acetyl Coa.
    - Thus PDHK-1 **blocks the forward direction of the TCA (TriCarboxylic Acid) cycle (also known as Kreb's cycle).**

- Thus pdhK pushes the cell to run on GLYCOLYSIS.

- **HIF causes increased glycolysis, and decreased Kreb's cycle** (in the forward direction).

- **Thus hypoxia can push the cell to running on glycolysis like a cancer cell!**

- HIF also induces increased secretion of **VEGF (Vascular Endothelial Growth Factor)** leading to **angiogenesis** — production of new blood vessels — that enables cancer cells to keep growing — and enables the cancer cells to metastasize!

- Prevent angiogenesis, and you prevent metastasis.

- Prevent hypoxia, and you might prevent angiogenesis.

- **Mutations** sometimes occur in the **enzymes** of **Kreb's cycle** called succinate dehydrogenase and fumarase making them less functional; which leads to accumulation of proximal, Kreb's cycle substrates like succinate and fumarate; which turn out to be inhibitors of **prolyl hydroxylase 2**.

- Normally, prolyl hydroxylase 2 functions to degrade HIF. When prolyl hydroxylase is inhibited by succinate and fumarate, that means that HIF 1 stays active.

- **Lactate accumulation** also inhibits prolyl hydroxylase 2, and thus prolongs the activation of HIF.

- Thus hypoxia alone can shift a cell into glycolysis based metabolism, and angiogenesis.

- Mutations in **Isocitrate DeHydrogenase** (IDH) lead to production of **2-hydroxy glutarate**.

- Normal enzyme isocitrate dehydrogenase converts isocitrate into alpha ketoglutarate.

- 2 hydroxy glutarate is considered an "onco-metabolite." 2 hydroxy glutarate **changes DNA methylation**, leading to the cell becoming **less dependent on growth factors**; in other words, the cell is **dedifferentiating**; going backwards in embryologic time;

    - backwards in evolutionary time; instead of being a functional part of an organ, that is a functional part of a human, the cell is now on its own;

    - just trying to grow independent of the adjacent cells.

- Insulin, insulin like growth factor, and estrogen are all growth factors.

- Normal cells only grow when get a signal from a growth factor that they should grow.

- **IDH mutation gets cells to grow even with relative lack of growth factors apparently.**

- There is evidence that if cancer cells can have electron transport & oxidative phosphorylation restored, the cancer cell might stop behaving like cancer, and restart to behave like a normal cell.

- Vitamin C helps to degrade HIF.
    - Vitamin C is an antioxidant that comes from plants.

OBESITY
- Fat people have increased sleep apnea which can lead to tissue hypoxia.
- Fatness is usually due to eating meat (animal protein + saturated fat), vegetable oils, and exposures to EDC's.

- **NIGHT SHIFT WORK.**
  - Body perceives lack of sleep as stress.
  - Chronic, excess psychological stress leads to chronic high cortisol.
  - Chronic high cortisol can damage neurons in the hippocampus, and lead to cognitive decline.
  - Messes up circadian rhythm.

Plant man Prometheus (Pmp): Do NOT be impressed by fancy statistics. Great treatments are obvious, and don't need fancy statistics. Fancy statistics are just a way to promote BS.

For example, populations who eat less than 300 mg per day of sodium, tend to NEVER develop hypertension even in their seventies. That's powerful information.

"Based on the inverse, square root, of the cosine of our data, we believe that this method has a relative risk improvement of 1.3." That's BS.

The things that matters most are "all cause mortality," and cognitive function.

All cause mortality is whether you live or die. That matters. Tumor shrinkage may or may not be significant. Cognitive impairment as a side effect of treatment is bad. You don't want that.

Skeptical Reader (SR): What causes cancer?

Veegus Rice (VR): **Cancer is primarily due to bad diet, and toxins, causing an abnormal microenvironment for cells.** Genetic vulnerabilities, DNA damage, and immunosuppression, increase the risk of cancer.

Vegan Prophet (VP):

Cancer is a renegade cell that has

de-evolved into behaving like a bacteria.

Pmp: An individual bacteria is not part of an organ system like the liver, pancreas, or colon. An individual bacteria just wants to grow for the sake of growth.

VP: Just like bacteria need iron to grow, cancer needs **iron** to grow. Cancer cells have a voracious appetite for iron. The immune system prevents cancer growth, by sequestering iron.

Normal human cells are part of organ systems, and perform their role in the organ.

Cancer cells are only out for themselves, and they grow uncontrollably, until they metastasize, and kill the patient.

Skeptical Reader (SR) How can a person improve their chances of living longer with cancer?

VP: Some foods – like MOFFUUC'S PP (Meat, Oil, Fluoride, industrial Fructose, Unknown additives, Unfiltered water, Processed food, Paleo – favor cancer growth. MOFFUUC'S PP eaters have about 5x as much cancer, as health vegans.

Some foods – like low fat, low sodium, organic, whole food, 100% vegan, no oil, no caffeine – favor normal cells.

Pmp: When normal cells of the organs, and the immune system are healthy, they make it hard for cancer to grow.

SR: Why do most people with cancer have mediocre outcomes?

Most people are mediocre, functional illiterates who think they are being smart, when they say stupid things.

SR: Examples please?

VP: They say things like, "I want the standard of care."

SR: What's wrong with that?

VP: The standard of care means the minimum level of care that must be provided to unconscious, intoxicated, and demented people.

An intelligent person, who is willing to read, should always want "OPTIMAL CARE."

SR: What's the difference between standard of care, and optimal care?

VP: Optimal care mostly means that the person does a lot on their own, to improve their health.

SR: What other mistakes do most people make?

VP: Most people try to apply "social ways" of thinking, to nutrition. That is a fatal mistake.

SR: What is the difference between social thinking, and nutritional thinking?

VP: Social thinking is linear. Middle of the pack is a safe place to be for social stuff. When in Rome, do as the Romans do. Go with the flow.

Nutritional thinking – for cancer prevention – is exponential. Cancer cells can amplify their number of cell surface – plasma membrane – receptors for growth factors.

If you give the cancer cell just a little bit of a tumor promoter – like meat, alcohol, tobacco, vegetable oil, estrogenic chemicals, iron – the cancer might start growing.

Skeptical reader: What can I do to decrease my risk of getting cancer? What can I do to increase my chance of surviving cancer?

Cancer is trying to kill you. Cancer is not your friend. F_ck cancer.

- **Exercise a lot**, because increases lymphatic flow 10-30x, which helps your immune system to remove cancer cells.

- Body fat makes estrogen; that's part of reason that fat women have more breast cancer.

- Increased sun exposure is associated with less risk of prostate cancer, and therefore probably lowers the risk of other cancers.

- **Do not give it one bite of meat.**[1] Meat increases Insulin Like Growth Factor (ILGF). ILGF increases cancer risk. The more fat you eat, the higher your risk of cancers like breast cancer,

---

1   "Experimental evidence of dietary factors and hormone dependent cancers." Cancer Res. 1975, Nov; 35 (11 pt2): 3374-83. Carroll. Lower calorie intake with less cancer. Higher dietary fat intake associated with increased cancer, especially breast cancer.

ovarian cancer, and prostate cancer. The more animal protein you eat, the higher your risk of cancer.[2] SAD diet is associated with increased cancer risk.

- Insulin – itself – is a "growth factor." Insulin is a mitogen. **Avoid things that cause insulin resistance.** Dietary fat causes insulin resistance. Potatos have only 1% fat. Low magnesium causes insulin resistance. Plants are a good source of magnesium.

- **Avoid sodium!** If you avoid processed foods, you will minimize your dietary sodium. Do not add sodium to your foods. Excess dietary sodium, and calcium – as well as a deficiency of dietary potassium and magnesium – all routine with the SAD diet – lead to increased cytoplasm calcium levels:

  - Increased cytoplasm calcium levels leads to increased insulin resistance;

  - Increased insulin resistance – which means resistance to skeletal muscle glucose uptake – leads to higher insulin levels in the blood;

  - the mitogenic effect of insulin remains relatively intact;

  - in other words – **excess ratio of dietary sodium and calcium to potassium and magnesium, leads to elevated insulin and MITOGENESIS!!!**[3] [4]

  - MITOGENESIS means increased cell division! You don't want increased mitogenesis in cancer cells!!

  - It's even worse than that. Elevated dietary sodium, leads to elevated cytoplasm calcium, and insulin resistance. Elevated cytoplasm calcium, and insulin resistance lead to the cell **PUMPING OUT PROTONS**; the cell pumps ACID into the extracellular matrix!!![5] [6]

    - This is the typical situation of a cancer cell. **Cancer cells gain an advantage over neighboring cells in an acidotic milieu!!**

  - Avoiding sodium mostly means avoiding Sodium Chloride which is abbreviated NaCl.

  - Dietary chloride is an anion, which means negatively charged ion. Excess dietary chloride displaces bicarbonate anion from the blood.

  - Bicarbonate is a pH buffer. When excess dietary chloride causes bicarbonate levels to go down, then the person develops a low grade ACIDOSIS.

  - The **low grade acidosis favors the growth of cancer cells.**

  - The low grade acidosis also kicks off cascades of metabolic problems like calcium leaching from the bones, calcium excretion in the kidneys coupled to pumping out protons into the urine to thus restore blood pH to normal; associated with calciuria; precpitation of calcium in kidney tubules; leading to kidney stones, and progressive kidney failure.

---

2 "The China study" book by T. Colin Campbell PhD, world famous expert on animal protein and cancer risk.
3 "The blood pressure solution" by Richard D. Moore MD PhD, copyright 1993.
4 "The insulin transduction system: a biophysical model for mitogenesis" Int'l Journal of quantum chemistry, quantum biol symp, 8 (1981): 365-371. Richard D Moore.
5 "Effects of insulin upon ion transport" Biochim biophys acta, 737:1-49 (1983) by Richard D. Moore.
6 "High blood pressure solution" by Richard D. Moore MD PhD, copyright 1993.

- And it's worse than that. The dietary induced metabolic acidosis leads to elevated cortisol levels which causes immune suppression, insulin resistance, and increased cancer risk.[7] [8]

- Excess sodium intake is especially associated with increased risk of gastric cancer (= stomach cancer) based on Japan, where sodium intake was high; high sodium intake in Japan was associated with increased risk of gastric cancer, and stroke.

- **NEVER eat nonorganic food.**[9] [10] [11] A commonly used herbicide in nonorganic food is associated in white blood cells (WBC's) – with possible DNA damage – to the p53 gene – that suppresses cancer; and damage to p53, might increase the risk of WBC cancers like lymphoma.[12]

- Not one drop of oil!

- Not one drop of alcohol! Alcohol is an evil spirit!

- Not one bite of meat!

- No iron supplements!

Starve the f_cker.

SR: Why so intense a response?

VP: I've studied cancer outcomes. The people who behave this way have the best outcomes. The most famous survivor is Ruth Heidrich PhD; you should read about her.

Pmp: You need to read to lead in outcomes. The goal is not to be in the middle of the pack with a "standard" outcome.

The goal is to have the 99.9% best possible outcome.

SR: What about all those people promoting the ketogenic and paleo diets for cancer?

VP: Dietary fat causes mitochondrial dysfunction. That has been shown by the extensive research on diabetes. The Michael Brownlee PhD paper makes that clear.

Dietary fat is another way of saying a meat based diet. Meat is the most powerful tumor promoter in the world.[13] [14]

Feeding meat to a cancer patient is insane.

---

7   "Acidosis is an old idea validated by research" Joseph Pizzomo, integr med 2015 Feb; 14(1): 8-12.
8   "Examining the relationship between diet induced acidosis and cancer." by Ian Forrest Robey. Nutrition and metabolism, 9, #72 (2012).
9   "Glyphosphate primes mammary cells for tumorigenesis by reprogramming the epigenome in a TET3-dependent manner" Frontiers in genetics (2019): 885, Manon Duforestel.
10 "Republished study: Long term toxicity of a… herbicide [glyphosphate] and … genetically modified maize" Environmental sciences Europe 26, (2014): 14. Gilles-Eric Seralini et al.
11 "Glyphosphate induces human breast cancer cells growth via estrogen receptors" Food and chemical toxicology 59 (2013):129-36. Thongprakaisang et al.
12 "DNA damage and methyulation induced by glyphosphate in human peripheral blood mononuclear cells" Food and Chem Toxicology 105, (2017), 93-98. Kwiatkowska et al.
13 "The China Study," 2005, by T. Colin Campbell PhD decribes data showing that meat promotes cancer.
14 "Dietary protein, growth factors, and cancer" Am J Clin nutr, June 2007. .

SR: What about a plant based, high fat diet?

VP: That won't work. David Blankenhorn, and others have shown that MUFA's (MonoUnsaturated Fatty Acids) – like olive oil – and PUFA's (PolyUnsaturated Fatty Acids) – are all about as atherogenic as saturated fat.

Things that cause atherosclerosis, cause less oxygen to tissues. Lowered oxygen delivery is called hypoxia. Hypoxia increases cancer risk, apparently because favors anaerobic metabolism, like cancer.

Fat is bad; bad, bad, bad!!! Run for your life. Avoid the fat. **There are no good fats.** Do not take fish oil. Fish oil potentially increases risk of prostate carcinoma, and of metastatic cancer, possibly due to immune suppression.[15] Omega 3 oils might also increase insulin resistance, causing increased insulin levels; not good; insulin is a mitogen; insulin stimulates cell replication.

Cancer cells have **cd36 sat fat receptors** especially for palmitic acid. Palmitic acid is C16:0, saturated fat). Palmitic acid is associated with increased risk of cancer.

Peter Rogers (PR): I do not do cancer research. I do not treat cancer patients. But I have read extensively about cancer pathophysiology, and outcomes.

Keto diet is high in animal protein, fat, sodium, iron. Keto diet promotes acidosis.

Sounds like a recipe to cause cancer.

I understand the rational, of trying to deprive cancer of glucose, but there are TOO MANY PROBLEMS with the keto diet.

Based on that reading, I can say, that Keto for cancer is one of the stupidest things I've ever heard. I believe it will accelerate the rate of death in cancer patients.

SR: Why is salt a risk factor for cancer?

VP: Sodium causes vasoconstriction, which causes tissue hypoxia.

The chloride in sodium chloride (table salt) is an anion (negatively charged ion). All bodily fluids have to balance their positive and negative ions. So when a person eats NaCl, the Cl- ions, displace the bicarbonate (HCO3-) ions.

HOC3- is a pH buffer. Addition of Cl- ions causes a low grade metabolic acidosis. Metabolic acidosis favors cancer growth.

SR: What is so good about plants?

VP: Plants contain high amounts of vasodilators like potassium, and magnesium. Vasodilators increase oxygen delivery to tissues. Good oxygen delivery, lowers cancer risk.

Plants contain vitamin C, and other antioxidants that help to repair DNA, and to prevent DNA damage. Prevention of mutations, helps to prevent cancer.

---

15   1. Griffini. **"Omega 3** fatty acids promote colon **carcinoma** metastases in rat liver." 1998, cancer res, aug 1;58(15)3312-19.
   2. Pelletier et al. "Influence of **lipid diets** on **metastases**." 1997, clin exp metastasis, Jul;15(4):410-17. 3. Klieveri.
   "**Promotion** of colon cancer **metastases** in rat liver by **fish oil diet**." 2000, clin exp metastasis, 2000; 18(5):371-77.

SR: Why is soda pop a risk factor for cancer?

The phosphoric acid can lead to a low grade metabolic acidosis. Soda pop often contains sodium chloride, to get the person to become thirstier; so they will buy more soda pop.

High fructose corn syrup, in soda pop, causes fatty liver. Fatty liver increases the risk of diabetes, and cancer.

Fatty liver is associated with higher blood lipids. Fructose is a LIPOGENIC sugar. Elevated blood lipids are associated with tissue hypoxia.

SR: Why is stress reduction so important?

VP: Stress increases cortisol and catecholamines. Cortisol suppresses the immune system. Your immune system is what protects you from cancer.

Catecholamines in high amounts cause insomnia. Your body heals during sleep. Insomnia causes increased cortisol. Catecholamines can function as siderophores – to transfer iron – to bacteria; maybe to cancer cells also? Don't want that.

Pmp: Stress also causes platelet activation. Platelet activation means to make the platelets more sticky, more prone to clotting.

SR: What is the significance of platelet activation?

VP: Platelet activation can cover metastatic cells, and hide them from the immune system.

Psychological stress – and stress equivalents like sleep deprivation, caffeine, loud noises – weaken your immune system.

SR: What about soy?

VP: Soy is too complicated. Soy is often processed in toxic ways with toxic solvents. Some doctors claim that soy increases ILGF (Insulin Like Growth Factor, a tumor promoter). Some researchers claim that soy is estrogenic, and goitrogenic. Some doctors and scientists claim that soy lowers risk of cancer. Like I was saying, it's too complicated to sort that out quickly. My advice is stay away from it.

SR: Can you just give me a list of how to optimize outcomes with cancer?

VP: Okay.

1. Read a lot about the thousands of people who have made great recoveries. You will learn from them. These are people were often at the brink of death, and survived. They will recommend the advice here, with lots of tips on how to reduce stress. If you have a smart family member, or friend, ask them to read these books. Single author books are the best. Two is the highest number of authors in great books. Whenever there are three or more authors, it ends up being a circle jerk, of lame-ola conformity, and defensive, wimpy, semi-illiterate prose. Read Dean Ornish, Ruth Heidrich, T. Colin Campbell, Chris Wark, "Radical Remissions" by Kelly Turner, and so on.

2. You want to spend as much time as possible in PANS, and as little as possible in SANS. PANS improves immune function.

3. Eat the low fat, low sodium, 100% plant based, whole food, vegan, organic diet.

4. Try to minimize your stress. Spend time with positive people. Try to be around people you love. Avoid negative people. Avoid petty people. Do not watch TV because it's stupid and negative. Comedy videos are okay.

5. Do something to help or be kind to someone else. Helping others energizes your immune system. I think that somehow, the unconscious mind senses that your life has value, and that you should be kept healthy. This lowers stress, and improves immune function.

6. Having a purpose in life makes you healthier.

7. Not one bite of meat. Never again in your life will you chew on an animal. The key to slowing cancer down, is to avoid tumor promoters. Meat is a tumor promoter in multiple ways.

8. Not one drop of milk. Milk is just a liquid form of meat. Milk is one of the most powerful cancer promoters in the world. World cancer expert, T. Colin Campbell claims that milk protein casein is the most powerful carcinogen in the world. No animal drinks milk after its been weaned. No animal drinks milk from another species. Neither should you.

9. Animal protein tends to be high in leucine. Leucine is the rate limiting step for activation of mTOR (mammallian Target Of Rapamycin). MTOR promotes cell growth and replication. You don't want that.

10. Methionine is an amino acid more common in meat. Methionine is an essential amino acid for some cancers; they can't grow without it. Deprive them of methionine, and the cancer's rate of growth, might decrease.

11. Meat is high in saturated fat. Sat fat causes RBC stiffening – decreased deformability – and RBC rouleaux which leads to tissue hypoxia. Hypoxia favors cancer growth.

12. Animal foods tend to be high in iron. Cancer has a voracious appetite for iron. Iron is a carcinogen. Do not eat anything with iron added to it.

13. Avoid sodium chloride (table salt). Sodium is a vasoconstrictor which causes tissue hypoxia. Tissue hypoxia favors cancer. Chloride is an anion (negatively charged ion). Chloride displaces bicarbonate ion out of the blood. Loss of bicarbonate ion buffer leads to a low grade acidosis. Acidosis favors cancer growth.

14. Not one drop of oil. Oil is a powerful tumor promoter. Do not eat any food if oil is one of the ingredients.

15. No junk food. No fast food. Junk food and fast food tend to be high in sodium, and contain toxic preservatives, and toxic emulsifiers, and toxic oil.

16. Only eat organic. Do not take one bite or one sip of nonorganic food. Nonorganic food routinely contains a herbicide that is considered a carcinogen.

17. The best foods do not even have a label, sweet potatos, potatos, carrots, and so on.

18. Not one drop of alcohol. Alcohol is a tumor promoter.

19. Not one puff of a cigarette. Tobacco is a tumor promoter.

20. Avoid foul smelling chemicals – like cleaning chemicals, glues, and paints – because they can be harmful to your health. They create extra work for your immune system. You want your immune system to be free to focus on removing the cancer.

21. Walk a lot, and consider jogging, or a stationary bike. Exercise increases flow in the lymphatic vessels. Good lymphatic flow improves immune system function.

22. Avoid endocrine disrupting chemicals. Reverse osmosis filter in your kitchen. Carbon filter for your entire house. Well water is usually better than city water, but you must test it to be sure of that. Do not drink fluoridated, chlorinated water. Do not put any chemicals on yourself: No deodorants. No laundry detergent. Minimize shampoo. No sunscreen. Almost anything you could put on your skin will have estrogen preservatives, like parabens. Estrogen preservatives increase the risk of breast cancer, endometrial cancer, and prostate cancer.

23. Consider donating blood to get your serum ferritin down to around 50. You need to get your blood labs checked first, so you know your baseline hemoglobin. You need to confirm with your doctor, that you don't have any contraindications to blood donation.

24. Do not take any supplements, unless there is a great reason. Routine multivitamins often contain iron which promotes cancer.

25. If your hobby makes you happy, then spend more time with that.

26. If religion makes you happy, then spend more time with that.

27. Good to have an attitude of gratitude. Gratitude improves immune function.

SR: What would you do if you had cancer?

PR: I would take some time off from work, so I could focus on optimizing my health, and reading.

I've already been reading about health optimization, and cancer prevention for years. I've already read lots of books by long term cancer survivors.

Newbies will need more time to read.

The same things that prevent cancer, will sometimes slow it's growth

I would become an expert on that particular type of cancer.

I would initially only talk to cancer doctors who were **NOT** going to treat me. I want objective opinions. If a doctor is part of a referral network, they have obligations to that network. That network has expectations of them — that they need to meet — to keep their jobs.

Luckily, I know lots of cancer doctors, so I could easily just talk to them.

If you don't know any, then read a lot first, and if you still need to talk to one, then figure out how to talk to one with no strings attached.

You could drive to another county, or another state.

The point is that you want OBJECTIVE opinions. You want to know the answer to questions like:

What percent of patients with this cancer are alive in 5 years, or 10 years? Does surgery, radiation, or chemo SIGNIFICANTLY increase survival.

I would only undergo an aggressive therapy if it was shown to generate a BIG increase in survival. You know that it is going to generate big side effects.

For example, testicular cancer tends to do well with chemo. Look at Lance Armstrong.

If the "improvement" in survival is small, then the side effects essentially cancel out the benefits.

I would not volunteer for any experimental research, because there will probably be side effects, and there are no proven benefits.

There is always some new treatment being hyped; and almost all of them fail. Avoid the hype.

I would find out if there is a blood test or imaging test to follow the tumor; for example, PSA (prostate specific antigen) is used to indicate risk of prostate carcinoma, and progression of prostate carcinoma.

I would try to optimize diet and life style, and see how that correlates with PSA, or whatever biomarker goes with the cancer type.

If the PSA was decreasing, I would assume I'm doing something right. If the PSA was going up, I would assume I was doing something wrong, and reassess diet and lifestyle.

If there weren't any great conventional treatments, then I would just try to optimize stuff on the list from this chapter.

I would try to minimize SANS and stress. SANS and stress weaken the immune system.

PANS strengthens the immune system. Therefore the more PANS, the better chance a patient has to prevent, and heal cancer.

It's your immune system that controls the cancer. It's your immune system that can cure you. I would do everything to strengthen my immune system. I would try to avoid anything that weakens my immune system.

SR: What about screening for cancer?

VP: Screening should only be done for high risk populations, like smokers.

Pmp: Low sodium, low fat, 100% plant based, organic, Vegans, with no oil, and no caffeine, and no alcohol, and no tobacco, are low risk for all cancers, as far as I know.

Low risk patient's do not need to screen. When low risk persons enter a screening study, they are much more likely to end up with false positives.

False positives can lead to prolonged, expensive, stressful, painful workups, with expensive, unnecessary surgery.

For every woman who "benefits" from mammography, lots more – at least twenty times more – suffer from worrying, unnecessary biopsies, etc.

By the time a breast cancer is seen on mammogram, the patient almost ALWAYS has metastases.[16] The best way to control metastases is to lower estrogen levels.[17] The best way to lower estrogen levels is to become a vegan, and to avoid all those estrogenic chemicals we talked about in this book, and in "Hot topics in nutrition," and on the you tube videos at "Peter Rogers MD."

The goal is to slow the rate of cancer growth. If you can slow it down enough, like a couple of decades, then you might be able to live, a long, healthy life.

SR: What do you actually do?

PR: I live by the list above in this chapter. My risk of cancer is very low. Therefore, I do not participate in any screening studies.

16 According to John McDougall MD, the best nutrition doctor in the world, and an expert on breast cancer.
17 According to John McDougall MD, the best nutrition doctor in the world, and an expert on breast cancer.

SR: What do your doctor friends do?

PR: The smartest doctors do what I do. The average doctors are only a small amount ahead of the general public in their health habits.

SR: Could you summarize your approach to cancer prevention?

PR: The healthcare system is designed to take care of SICK people. Healthy people do not need the system.

The best option for smart people – which means the top 1 or 2 percent – is to optimize ALL their habits, so that they stay healthy.

SR: Why do you limit this to the top 1 or 2%? Shouldn't that be the best option for all people?

PR: Ha, ha, ha. I have lots of doctor friends, and most of them eat meat, and oils, and many of them are overweight.

They are NOT healthy. It's not even possible to get most doctors to be healthy.

Optimal health is only for health aristocrats; people with the ability to read, and change their behavior. 30 years of being a doctor has taught me that this is about 1-2% of the population.

SR: But higher percentages of people have optimal habits in other countries, like Okinawa.

PR: Herd animals copy the herd. Corporations set the pattern for the herd. Corporations want the herd fat and sick, so they can make money off the herd.

A fat man and his money are soon parted.

No one makes money off skinny vegans.

Chapter 6

Female problems and Estrogen

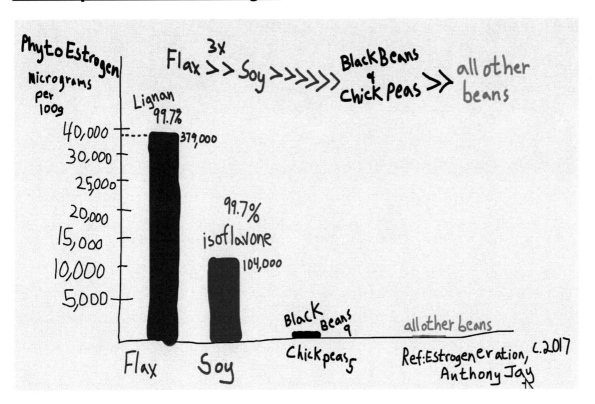

Fig 104: **Flax has an incredibly high amount of estrogen**, even more than soy. Soy is thousands of times more estrogenic than most foods.

What problems are caused by (or associated with) high estrogen levels?

- Dysfunctional uterine bleeding with long periods.

- Menstrual cramps.

- PMS.

- Endometriosis.

- Morning sickness of pregnancy.

- Postpartum depression.

- Obesity.

- Fibroids.

- Adenomyosis of the uterus = endometrial-glandular tissue in the myometrial -muscle layer of the uterus.

- Increased risk autoimmune diseases.

- Increased risk post menopausal hot flashes.

- Increased benign breast masses, like fibrocystic disease.

- Increased risk breast cancer.

- Increased risk endometrial cancer.

Why do so many woman have high estrogen levels?

- Eating meat.

    - Because the liver conjugates estrogen with another chemical, and then excretes it into the bile.

    - Normally, women poop out their extra estrogen.

    - Meat changes gut bacteria.

    - Meat based gut bacteria have the enzyme "glucoronidase" to deconjugate estrogen.

    - This deconjugated estrogen is then reabsorbed from the gut, back into the blood.

- Drinking whole milk.

    - Nowadays, the milk cow is usually engineered to produce milk while it's pregnant.

    - Pregnant cows have very high estrogen levels.

    - Pregnant cow, extra estrogen, gets into the milk.

- Drinking water that contains estrogens.

    - Municipal water filtration often does not remove estrogens well;

    - like EE2 (Ethinyl Estradiol of birth control pills) and atrazine (herbicide).

    - Yes. Your tap water might contain EE2, and atrazine.

- Storing drinks in BPA, or other estrogenic containers.

    - Just because the container says, "no BPA," it might be a BPA substitute like BPS, which is still estrogenic.

    - Watch out for cans. The lining of cans often is made with BPA.

- Cosmetic skin products with estrogenic preservatives like the parabens.

- Soaps and shampoos with estrogen. I use the safest of newborn baby shampoos, and it still contains an estrogenic.

- Laundry detergents with estrogen.

    - A typical detergent is nonoxynol-9, an estrogen.

    - The plastic container is often made out of BPA, and pthalates, which are both estrogenic.

    - That's three estrogens on your "clean" clothes.

    - All day long, these clothes contact your skin, and estrogen is absorbed through your skin, and into your blood.

What else can a woman do to normalize her estrogen levels?

- Avoid meat and milk.

- Do not put cosmetic products on her skin; especially avoid aluminum deodorant.

  - We greet each other by saying, "Hello."

  - We do not sniff each other's armpits.

  - If you are a low IQ, wimpy conformist who insists on wearing deodorant, then at least do NOT shave your pits.

  - Shaving increases transdermal absorption.

- Wash clothes without detergent. Just run the washer and dryer longer and hotter.

- Store beverages in glass.

- Obtain a carbon filter, or reverse osmosis filter for water.

What's the key concept for understanding estrogen disrupting chemicals (EDC's)?

Estrogen, the hormone, for millions of years, in the animal kingdom, had no competition.

Estradiol is the main form of estrogen. The active part of the estradiol molecule is the "phenol group."

A phenol group is a hydroxy group attached to a benzene. The benzene ring is also called an aromatic ring because it gives off an "aroma."

Benzene rings are cyclohexanes with three double bonds that resonate; this resonance confers super stability; this stuff can sit on a shelf for years, and remain unchanged.

The hydroxy group (phenol group) confers antimicrobial activity.

Do you get it?

Estrogenic chemicals, like parabenzoic acid, are the **PERFECT PRESERVATIVE**; long shelf life, and antimicrobial.

That's why EDC's (Estrogen Disrupting Chemicals) are almost always put into skin care products.

That's why I recommend to **avoid all skin care products**.

What should people do with their cosmetic products?

In the 1490's Girolamo Savanarola called for a **BONFIRE OF THE VANITIES**.

It is time to call for a bonfire of cosmetic vanities.

If women want to burn their bras too, men won't complain.

Just kidding. You don't need to burn your cosmetics — that would create toxic smoke — but you should throw most of that junk into the garbage.

Why do these chemicals have an estrogenic effect?

The estrogen receptor simply recognizes the "phenol group" component of the molecule for activation. The estrogen receptor doesn't care much what is attached to the phenol group.

During the millions of years during which the estrogen receptor was "evolving," these other chemicals did not exist.

The estrogen receptor is a bit of a "slut." Just show her a phenol group, and she will open up, and hydrogen bond with it, and get activated.

What happens when the estrogen receptor gets activated?

Estrogen causes proliferation of breast cells, and endometrial cells.

Excess estrogen, and EDC's can lead to excess proliferation of breast, and endometrial cells, with resultant cancer.

Where can one learn more about estrogen biochemistry, and disease avoidance?

In my other book, "How to prevent cancer and chronic disease," I go into much more detail about estrogen physiology, and which products, and preservatives are estrogenic.

What about PCOS?

PCOS is Poly Cystic Ovary Syndrome. PCOS has several causes: genetic vulnerability, obesity, diabetes, and potentially elevated intracranial pressure (as it relates to CSF pressure theory).

Obesity and diabetes are asssociated with a decrease in steroid hormone binding globulin (SHBG).

Normally, SHBG binds to androgens and estrogens in the blood. When blood levels of SHBG are lowered, then there is more "free" estrogen and androgen going around causing problems.

What's the benefit of low fat, low salt, vegan diet for PCOS?

Optimizes body weight, so that obesity goes away, and diabetes might go away, and SHBG levels increase.

Avoiding exogenous estrogenics like BPA, aluminum, nonoxynol 9, parabens and so on, can help for treatment of PCOS.

Only eat organic foods. Nonorganic food is more likely to have residues from estrogenic herbicides like atrazine.

Here's a little verse to keep it terse:

- Estrogenics make you fat and SICK.

- They hide in lotion and PLASTIC.
- Go through your skin like MAGIC.

- Feminization of frogs and FISHES,
- Messes up her cycle.
- Turns Betties into BITCHES.

- Woman got no baby.
- Man got no D_CK.

- Molecular memory, it's real SLICK.
- Autoimmune and ALLERGIC.

- Now we know their little TRICK,
- We gonna avoid them real QUICK.

The inspiration for the above poem was the lovely childhood rhyme I learned in 7th grade when the girls were skipping rope and singing:

- "Ding, dong, you're momma don'na wear no drawers.

- I saw her when she took'em off.

- She laid them on the table.

- Them fruits ain't got no flava."

Chapter 7

Lipids and oils and bears, oh my!

All fat is bad. There are no good fats. The only dietary fat you need, is the minimal amount present in low fat, plant foods. Even omega 3 fats are associated with increased risk of prostate cancer.

The so called "good fats" are metabolic poisons. Fallen angel number one is olive oil. Olive oil carries a lot of emotional baggage. Odysseus and Penelope built their marriage bed around an olive tree.[18]

I love the Greeks. I love the Italians. But olive oil has no place in a healthy diet.

Olive oil is all hype, and no real benefit. Look at the name, "Extra Virgin Olive Oil." That sounds like marketing for romance.

The "Mediterranean diet" is a bogus concept.   People just use the phrase "Mediterranean diet" as an excuse to eat fish, olive oil, wine, cheese, eggs, chicken, and other metabolic poisons.

Olive oil, like all oils, is liquid fat. Liquid fat has no nutrients. All dietary fat promotes obesity.

Olive oil, like all oils, is thought to be toxic to your gut lining (enterocytes), your red blood cells (rouleaux formation), your platelets (increaed stickiness), your arterial lining (endothelium), and your skeletal muscle (insulin resistance).[19]

In general, vegetable oils contain a lot of omega six fats: safflower, sunflower, soybean oil, corn oil, and cottonseed oil are all 50-80% omega 6 fat, especially, linoleic acid 18:2.

Skeptical Reader (SR): What about those doctors who publicly have said that olive oil is "heart healthy?"

VP (Vegan Prophet): What food companies do, is they rig short term studies by making olive oil part of a moderately healthy diet, and then comparing it to a very poor diet.

SR: On what evidence do you condemn olive oil?

VP: First of all, let's talk about its scientific name. The main type of fat in olive oil is oleic acid, with its deprotonated form called "oleate."

Oleate is a C18 fatty acid, meaning that it has 18 carbons. Oleate is a monounsaturated fatty acid (MUFA), meaning that it has one double bond. Oleate is the most common MUFA in nature.

Oleate is written as C18:1, delta 9 which means that the 18 carbon fatty acid, has a single double bond, on carbon number 9.

Pmp (Plant Man Prometheus): By the way, olive oil routinely contains about 13% saturated fat, especially palmitate, C16:0. By that alone, I would never eat it.

Olive oil is also about 10% composed of an omega 6 fat called Lin-Oleic acid, C18:2. Omega 6 fats are proinflammatory. Lin-oleic acid is a PUFA (PolyUnsaturated Fatty Acid).

---

18 **Penelope** questioned **Oddyseus** about the olive tree to confirm his identity, when he returned after twenty years, in the *Oddysey*.

19 Silva et al. "Olive, soybean, palm oil have similar acute detrimental effect on endothelial function in healthy young subjects" Nutr Metab Cardiovasc dis 2007;17:50.

VP: Robert Vogel MD is a famous cardiologist who has pioneered a brachial artery tourniquet test to show endothelial function.[20]

The tourniquet is placed on the upper arm for 5 minutes, and then released. Transcutaneous ultrasound then measures the diameter of the brachial artery.

Pmp: The tourniquet time causes ischemia of the forearm. Therefore – when the tourniquet is released – a normal brachial artery will vasodilate – enlarge in diameter – to permit more blood flow to the forearm. The endothelial cells release nitric oxide – vasodilator – which causes the artery to dilate.

Healthy arteries are dynamic; they vasoconstrict (narrow), and vasodilate (widen), in response to local tissue, oxygen needs.

VP: However, when endothelial cells are injured by dietary fat, they are less able to make nitric oxide.

Olive oil decreased the brachial artery's ability to dilate by 31%.

All dietary fat has a negative effect on blood flow which is worst at 3 to 6 hours postprandial.[21]

Pmp: Dietary olive oil also increases the tendency of RBC's to develop rouleaux formation.

Dietary fat increases insulin resistance, and the risk of diabetes.

VP: Salad dressing is for puzzies. You don't need it. I eat my salads plain, like a manly man.

SR: What about oils for cooking?

Pmp: You don't need oils for cooking. Up until about 100 years ago, people cooked without oils.

For most starches, all you need to do is boil water: beans, potatos, sweet potatos, rice, oatmeal, quinoa.

Most fruits and vegetables are eaten raw: carrots, blueberries, apples, pears, bananas, salad.

VP: Oils are the "Achilles heel" of philosophical vegans.[22] [23]

Pmp: I have an Indian doctor friend, who is quite skinny. I did not see him for a couple of months. Upon seeing him again, I said, "Where have you been?"

Indian doctor friend (Idf): I died, but I'm okay now.

Pmp: What?

Idf: I had a heart attack, and coded, but they successfully resuscitated me, and they put in a coronary artery stent.

Pmp: I thought you were a vegetarian.

Idf: I am.

Pmp: It must be oils! Do you put oil in your food?

Idf: Oh yeah. You need that for cooking.

20 "Postprandial effects of components of Mediterranean diet on endothelial function." Robert Vogel et al. J am coll cardiology, vol 36, no 5, 2000. Olive oil caused reduced dilation of brachial artery, indicating decreased function of endothelical cells, and decreased nitric oxide production.
21 Angina pectoris induced by fat ingestion in pt's with coronary artery disease." Peter Kuo MD, JAMA 1955 July. Great paper. Chest pain occurred at peak lipemia at about 5 hours. Peak lipemia was at about 4-6 hours!! Therefore after a high fat meal, a person has high blood lipids from at about 2-8 hours.
22 Takahash et al. "High MUFA diet induced obesity & diabetes in mice" Metabolism 1998, Jun; 47 (6): 724.
23 Wilson et al. "Dietary MUFA's promote atherosclerosis in mice" Arterioscler Thromb Vasc Biol. 1998; 18; 1818.

Pmp: No, you don't. All oils are bad for health, and that includes olive oil, coconut oil, and fish oil.

VP: Whenever I hear that a 100% vegan has coronary artery disease, it's usually due to dietary oil.[24] [25] [26] Atherosclerosis worsens just as much from MUFA as from saturated fat.

Pmp: Caldwell Esselstyn MD has the best results in the world for the prevention of coronary artery disease. Esselstyn's diet is 100% plant based, with no oils, no nuts, and no caffeine.

Esselstyn's results are about 40 times better than those obtained with a version of the Mediterranean diet.[27] [28]

VP: When you look closely at the data, it becomes obvious that any intelligent person would choose the Vegan diet over drugs, stents, or surgery.

Pmp: In the health care world,

it is ASTONISHING how few people read.

99.9% of people choose drugs, stents, surgery over the Vegan diet,

and they pay a high price for their ignorance.

VP: We already talked about coronary artery disease in the chapter on that subject. But to briefly summarize: elective stenting and CABG have only a minimal benefit, and usually do not decrease the risk of future myocardial infarction, or all cause mortality.

Pmp: High tech is great for computers, and great for radiology machines, but the human body prefers low tech approaches like diet and exercise.

Ding dong! The old monarchs of stents and surgeries are dead!

Long live the new monarchs of Vegan diet and exercise!

SR: Hold on a second. **Interventional cardiologists save lots of lives by reopening arteries during acute myocardial infarctions (MI).**

VP: Yes. For acute MI, cardiac cath with stent placement saves lives.

Pmp: But most patients have chronic symptoms.

SR: And cardiac surgery saves lots of lives.

VP: Yes. There are some patients who greatly benefit from cardiac surgery. Cardiac patients are often complex, with combined arterial, and valvular disease.

Pmp: Granted. There are a lot of patients who benefit from stents, and surgery. However, **the VAST MAJORITY of patients would obtain optimal results by becoming health vegans.**

24 Blankenhorn et al. "Influence of diet on the appearance of new lesions in human coronary arteries" Jama, 1990; 263(12):1646. Atherosclerotic plaques progressed just as much eating a diet high in MUFA's as a diet high in sat fat.
25 Rudel et al. "Compared with dietary MUFA & sat fat, PUFA protects African green monkeys from coronary artherosclerosis" Arterioscl thromb vasc biol. 1995;15:2101.
26 "Effects of dietary fat on postproandial activation of blood coagulation factor 7" Arterioscler thromb vasc biol, 1997, Nov; 17 (11) 2904. Larsen et al
27 Esselstyn et al." A way to reverse CAD? J Fam Practice. 2014;63:356-364.
28 "Prevent and reverse heart disease" book by Caldwell Esselstyn MD.

In a health vegan population – following an Esselstyn equivalent diet – coronary artery disease does not exist.

Obesity does not exist.

VP: When one also makes the diet "low sodium," then hypertension usually does not exist.

Pmp: And when eating plant foods, there is adequate potassium, and magnesium, and fiber; so cognitive function is improved, and abdominal pressure syndrome is minimized, and autoimmune disease is rare.

Paradise regained!

VP: You only get one life on this planet. Make it healthy. Choose Vegan: the only diet proven to prevent atherosclerosis, obesity, hypertension, and diabetes.

SR: What about the difference between grass fed cattle versus factory farm cattle?

VP: Yeah, sure. Factory farm cattle that are fed a diet high in omega 6 fats, are going to have more omega 6 fats.

But the point is moot. People should not eat any meat. You can't polish a turd. Meat is a metabolic poison. Even the best possible meat is high in animal protein and saturated fat; poison for humans.

The only exception is human breast milk, during infancy. That's it.

SR: How much fat is ideal for adult humans?

VP: Less than 5%. Ideally, I would like my dietary fat to be about 5%, but that's hard to achieve.

A low fat, low sodium, 100% plant based, starch based diet will probably lead to about 10% fat, 10% protein, and 80% carbohydrate.

Kempner's rice diet was about 5% fat, 5% protein, and 90% carbohydrate.

The lower that fat content, the skinnier the population; the lower the cancer rates.

Pmp: Most people do not know that meat has tons of fat, especially saturated fat. Butter is about 55% sat fat. Beef has about 50% sat fat. Pork has about 40% sat fat. Chicken has about 30% sat fat.

SR: How does fatty acid nomenclature work?

VP: Fatty acids are long chain carboxylic acids. In organic chemistry nomenclature, numbering of fatty acid carbons begins with the carbonyl carbon (also known as the carboxylic carbon). The carboxylic acid is polar. The fatty acid "tail" is nonpolar, hydrophobic.

In the biochemistry and nutritional literature, the numbering begins with the METHYL end carbon which is also called the OMEGA end. The METHYL method is better for nutrition and biochemistry because the omega end remains constant. With the METHYL method, when there is an elongation reaction, the double bond stays in the same numerical place; like for making a C18:3, w-3 fatty acid, into a longer fatty acid, like EPA C20:5, or DHA C22:6.

The "w" designation is for the location of the double bond, based on counting from the METHYL end carbon, which is also called the OMEGA end carbon.

SR: What is saturated fat?

VP: Saturated fat has no double bonds. Saturated fat is usually solid at room temperature. Butter is a good example of saturated fat. The fat in steak is primarily saturated fat.

Saturated fat causes a big increase in LDL cholesterol, which is quite atherogenic. Saturated fat accumulation in RBC plasma membranes, causes stiffening of those membranes. Stiff RBC membranes means increased blood viscosity.

Increased blood viscosity means increased blood pressure. Increased blood pressure means increased atherosclerosis. Increased atherosclerosis means increased myocardial infarction.

SR: What are common examples of saturated fat?

C16:0 is palmitic acid. PALMitic acid is the most common form of saturated fat. PALMitic oil is of course very common in PALM oil. Palmitic is also the most common type of saturated fat in beef, chicken, pork, and milk.

C18:0 is stearic acid. Stearic acid is the second most common form of saturated fat.

SR: What about omega 3 fats?

VP: Omega 3 fats have a double bond at the number 3 position, which is listed as w-3.

SR: What are common examples of omega 3 fats?

VP: C18:3 w-3 is alpha linoleNic acid (ALA) which is present in plant foods.

C20:5 w-3 is EPA (EicosaPenaenoic Acid); especially present in ocean plants, and cold water fish.

C22:6 w-3 is DHA (DocosaHexaenoic Acid); especially present in ocean plants, and cold water fish.

SR: Why do all the common fatty acids have an even number of carbons?

VP: Because they are built up from 2 carbon units, called acetyl units. Palmitic acid C16:0 is the most common fatty acid, made in mammals, by fatty acid synthase.

SR: Are omega 3 fats good for you?

VP: No. Omega 3 fats are still an oil. All oils are bad for health. It is difficult to purify fish oil, and there is concern about risk of contamination.[29] [30] [31]

Pmp: Omega 3 oil is a highly processed food. All oils promote obesity.

VP: Increased dietary omega 3 oil is associated with possible increased insulin resistance and diabetes, and possibly increased risk of prostate cancer.

SR: What are common examples of omega 6 fats?

VP: C18:2 w-6 is Linoleic acid.

SR: What are common examples of MUFA's (MonoUnsaturated Fatty Acids)?

VP: C18:1 w-9 is oleic acid. Oleic acid is the main type of oil in olive oil, comprising about 73% of olive oil.

SR: What other oils are found in olive oil?

VP: It depends on the type of olive oil. Olive oil may contain saturated fat like palmitic oil up to at least 11%, and omega 6 oil like Linoleic acid C18:2 w-6, up to 9%, and omega 3 fat like alpha linolenic acid up to .8%.[32] Notice that these numbers show a significant amount of saturated fat, and a ratio of omega 6 fat >> omega 3 fat.

29 "Dietary PUFAS and composition of human aortic plaques." Lancet, 1994, Oct 29, 344 (8931): 1195.
30 "Dietary fat intake and early age related lens opacities" Am j clin jutr. 2005, Apr; 81 (4):773. Gail Rogers et al. Increased dietary inatke of C18 PUFA's linoleic acid and linolenic acid was associated with increased risk of cataracts.
31 Griffini, P. "Dietary omega 3 PUFA's promote colon carcinoma metastases in rat liver." Cancer res, 1998, Aug 1; 58 (15) 3312
32 "Advanced nutrition and Human metabolism" book by Sareen Gropper p. 129.

SR: What is the significance of the omega 6 to omega 3 ratio?

VP: Our ancestors are thought to have eaten a ratio of omega 6 to omega 3 of about 1:1. Nowadays, MOFFUUC'S PP eaters get a huge excess of omega 6 fats >>> omega 3; and this causes inflammation.

SR: What is a triglyceride?

VP: Triglycerides (TG's) are also called TriAcyl Glycerides (TAG's). Acyl means fatty acid group, as in fatty acid being part of a larger molecule, like a TAG.

Glycerol is the "backbone" of TAG's. Glycerol is the same thing as "propane-triol," which is a 3 carbon alkane with a hydroxyl group – (hydroxyl group is same thing as an alcohol group) – on each carbon.

The vast majority of dietary fat is triglycerides. When someone says "fat," they usually mean triglyceride, unless otherwise specified.

SR: What is the difference between a fatty acyl group, and a free fatty acid?

VP: An "acyl group" usually refers to a fatty acid group on a bigger molecule, like a TAG.

A free fatty acid is by itself. Free fatty acids are sometimes called NEFA's (Non-Esterified Fatty Acids). Most fatty acids in the typical fat person, are in storage form, which means esterified to a glycerol molecule, as part of a TAG, in adipose tissues.

SR: What determines the solubility of a fatty acid?

VP: Saturated fatty acids tend to be solid at room temperature, because their carbon tails have a standard, monotonous, up and down pattern, that enables them to interdigitate closely, with each other.

Double bonds are normally in cis configuration. Cis double bonds cause a BIG BEND in the carbon tail. This big bend "pushes away" other fatty acids – like in a plasma membrane fatty acid bilayer – so that the membrane is "fluidized."

The more double bonds, the more likely the fatty acid is oil = liquid.

The longer the fatty acid – ie. the more carbons in the tail – the more likely it is solid.

The effect of double bonds can "overpower" the effect of fatty acid length; EPA and DHA are liquid at body temperature. That's how "fish oil" helps prevent the fish from freezing in cold temperatures.

SR: What is a phospholipid?

VP: A phospho-lipid contains phosphate and lipid. The phosphate is just a phosphate. The lipid is a Di-Acyl Glycerol. Phospholipids are the second most common type of dietary fat.

Pmp: Di-Acyl Glycerol (DAG) + Phosphate is called **Phospha-Tidic Acid (PTA)**. PTA is the "building block" for most phospholipids.

Membrane phospholipids are made by starting with PTA and adding a "head group" like choline, or serine, or inositol, or ethanolamine.

For example: PhosphaTidic Acid + Choline = PhosphaTidyl Choline. PhosphaTidyl Choline is the most common membrane phospholipid in mammals.

SR: What is CARDIOLIPIN?

VP: Cardiolipin is a unique fatty acid. Cardiolipin is a "giant size" phospholipid. Cardiolipin consists of 2 PTA's connected by a glycerol. Cardiolipin is mostly found in the inner mitochondrial membrane.

The fatty acid tails on cardiolipin are often PUFA's. The fact that cardiolipin has several PUFA type fatty acid tails, and it is located on the inner mitochondrial membrane – the hot spot in the human body for the production of reactive oxygen, free radicals – makes it obvious that cardiolipin is highly vulnerable to lipid peroxidation!![33]

SR: What about lipid peroxidation?

VP: Lipid peroxidation is a major problem with PUFA's (PolyUnsaturated Fatty Acids). A PUFA is any fatty acid with two or more double bonds.

A methylene group is a CH2 group. The methylene bridge carbon – the single bonded carbon, between a pair of double bonds – has only a "weak" grip on its hydrogen – and is vulnerable to lipid peroxidation.

Lipid peroxidation is a chain reaction that progresses like a stack of dominoes, to destroy lots of other lipids.

Lipid peroxidation can be very damaging to plasma membranes, and to mitochondrial membranes. Cardiolipin is especially vulnerable to lipid peroxidation. The brain has a relatively large amount of PUFA's in its cell membranes, and this makes the brain more vulnerable to oxidative stress, and lipid peroxidation.

Pmp: With lipids, there's always more details to talk about.

VP: The key point is to **minimize dietary lipids!** There are no "good fats." **FAT IS BAD!** The way to minimize dietary lipids is to eat a low fat, plant based diet.

SR: What is the difference between cholesterol and a steroid?

VP: Cholesterol has 4 rings of carbon – labeled A, B, C, D – and a total of 27 carbons. Cholester-OL has a hydroxy group at the C3 position (on the A ring).

The steroid nucleus also has 4 rings of carbon, based on the 4 rings of cholesterol.

SR: How does the steroid nucleus relate to steroid hormones, and estrogen?

VP: In general, the steroid hormones are made by starting with cholesterol, then removing the alkane chain attached to C17, then adding some hydroxy groups, alcohol groups, or ketones.

SR: Why is estrogen unique?

VP: Estrogen is unique, because it's the only one with a benzene ring. The A ring of estrogen is a "benzene."

SR: What is the characteristic feature of bile acids?

VP: Like the name says, the **bile ACIDS** are based on an ACID. To make a **primary bile ACID**, a **carboxylic acid** is added to a **cholesterol** molecule. Then a couple of hydroxyl groups are added. Primary bile acids are made in the liver.

This combination of nonpolar (hydrophobic), and polar (hydrophilic) regions, enables bile acids to function as **EMULSIFIERS**, for digestion of fats.

Pmp: The liver then "conjugates" the primary bile acids. **Conjugation** consists of **adding an amino acid** to the bile acid. Typically, **glycine or taurine** is added to the primary bile acid. The new chemical is called a **"conjugated" bile acid.**

SR: What about bile salts?

---

33 Douglas Kell. "**Iron behaving badly**." 2009. Great paper! Douglas Kell is a from England and he is the most entertaining speaker on the topic of iron metabolism. He claims that excess, unliganded-free iron can cause an autocatalytic chain reaction of reactive oxygen species via Fenton and Haber Weiss reactions leading to cellular death from lipid peroxidation (cell membrane damage) and DNA damage. He also claims that excess free iron can "reawaken" dormant bacteria. This paper has an interesting diagram of iron metabolism.

VP: The conjugated bile acid becomes deprotonated, so it carries a negative charge. The negative charge attracts a positive charge. Ions like sodium and potassium will bind to the deprotonated bile acid. The combination of deprotonated bile acid combined with sodium or potassium is called a **bile salt.**

Pmp: The terms bile acid and bile salt are often used interchangeably.

SR: What happens to the bile acids?

VP: About 95% of bile acids are reabsorbed – mostly in the ileum. The reabsorbed bile salts travel through the portal vein so they can return to the liver.

SR: What about secondary bile acids?

VP: Some gut bacteria in the colon will remove a "hydroxyl group," from a conjugated primary bile acid, at carbon number seven.

The resultant molecule is called a **"secondary" bile acid.**

SR: What is the significance of secondary bile acids?

VP: Secondary bile acids are unique in the sense that they are in the **COLON**. The **higher** the concentration of **secondary bile acids** in the colon, the **higher** the risk of **colon cancer.**[34]

Pmp: The **MORE FAT A PERSON EATS, THE MORE BILE GETS SECRETED**; and the more bile reaches the colon; and the more colon cancer.

Rvw: Rural Africans who eat a plant based diet **hardly ever get colon cancer**. African Americans commonly get colon cancer.

This is old information. Denis Burkitt and Nathan Pritikin knew all this stuff about fiber and colon cancer back in the 1960's and 1970's.

SR: Why does meat increase the risk of colon cancer?

VP: Meat increases the risk of colon cancer because:

1. **High fat** content leads to **MORE SECONDARY BILE ACIDS** in colon. All dietary fat – beyond the small amount in low fat plant foods – is bad for the colon. Even PUFA's (PolyUnsaturated Fatty Acids) cause increased risk of colon carcinoma in animal studies.

2. High fat associated with insulin resistance, and higher insulin levels, and i**nsulin is a growth factor.**

3. Meat leads to higher blood levels of insulin like growth factor (**ILGF**).

4. Meat has no fiber. Lack of fiber leads to proliferation of **bad gut bacteria**.

5. Promotion of bad gut bacteria that produce hydrogen sulfide, and are associated with inflammatory bowel disease.

6. Saturated fat leads to RBC rouleaux, and relative **hypoxia** of tissues.

7. Increased Polycyclic Aromatic Hydrocarbons (**PAH**).

8. Increased herbicides.

9. Increased pesticides.

10. Increased antibiotics in the meat which kills good gut bacteria.

11. Increased estrogen.

12. Increased **N-Nitroso compounds**.

---

34 "Fat, fibre, and cancer risk in African Americans, and rural Africans" Nat commun, Apr 2015, 6:6342.

13. Increased **TMAO**.

14. Increased sulfur containing amino acids like methionine, and cysteine with resultant low grade metabolic acidosis.

15. Increased AGE's.

16. Increased **Heterocyclic Aromatic Amines**.

17. Increased atherosclerosis which can lead to tissue hypoxia.

Chapter 8

Is organic worth it?

Some of the absolute, best, nutrition doctors in the world like Caldwell Esselstyn MD and John McDougall MD do NOT emphasize organic. Some of the most famous hospitals in the world have health newsletters, and they do NOT emphasize organic.

They are wrong.

They say that while organic is preferable to nonorganic, the most important thing is that people eat 100% plant foods.

I agree that eating plant foods is the most important thing, but I've studied the herbicides and pesticides in nonorganic foods.

There appear to be major toxicities from the pesticides and herbicides in nonorganic foods – according to books and research studies – and you should avoid them if possible.[35] [36]

Are poor people fated to poor health?

If you go to the grocery store in a lower middle class, or poor neighborhood, there is hardly any organic food. This means that poor people are exposed to more herbicides and pesticides in their foods.

Cheap, subsidized foods often contain a lot of salt (sodium chloride) which increases risk for hypertension, atherosclerosis, myocardial infarction (heart attack), stroke, kidney failure (dialysis), and kidney stones.

Poor people often drink tap water, without any water filter. Unfiltered tap water often contains multiple estrogenic chemicals like atrazine, and so on, which are associated with obesity, diabetes, hypertension, breast cancer, and prostate cancer.

Poor people often work in factory jobs, or janitorial jobs, or automotive jobs, (like driving a bus) where they are exposed to toxic chemicals.

Poor people have more financial stress which can cause psychological stress.

What is organic?

Organic farms are supposed to undergo – annual on site inspections – by the USDA – to insure they are following the organic guidelines.

The main guidelines include no GMO, and many herbicides and pesticides are forbidden.

Is all organic food okay?

Of course not. There are lots of organic junk foods like fried, organic, potato chips, and sweets.

Can organic contain MSG?

Yes. MSG means MonoSodium Glutamate. Glutamate is a naturally occurring amino acid, and therefore is allowed in organic foods.

Lots of organic foods have MSG added.

How can MSG be avoided?

---

35   Toxic Legacy" by Stephanie Seneff, copyright 2021.
36   "Food Forensics: the hidden toxins lurking in your food, and how you can avoid them for lifelong health" by Mke Adams

Learn the many "names" of MSG, and avoid them. MSG is often hidden under the name of "extract," or "natural flavors."

Only eat single ingredient foods. Sometimes MSG is "hidden" in secondary ingredients.

Can organic contain GMO?

USDA organic certified foods are not allowed to contain GMO (Genetically Modified Organisms) food.

What herbicides are forbidden with organic?

USDA certified foods are not allowed to contain atrazine or glyphosphate.[37]

There is concern that some of the herbicides in nonorganic food are associated with increased risk of lymphoma, which is a type of cancer.[38]

What about pesticides?

Nonorganic foods overall, tend to have more pesticide residues.

Organophosphate pesticides are thought to increase the risk of Parkinson's disease.

Does organic forbid human sludge as fertilizer?

Yes. Organic forbids human feces as fertilizer.

If a food is labeled "Non-GMO," does that mean there's no glyphosphate on it?

No. Glyphosphate is sometimes used as a "dessicant" on non-gmo foods like wheat, barley, rye, oats, peas, garbanzo beans (chick peas), and lentils. The glyphosphate causes the plant to shed its leaves, so it's easier to harvest. Other crops potentially sprayed with glyphosphate include sunflower seeds.[39]

According to some authors, glyphosphate is especially used as a dessicant in colder countries, like Canada, because they have a shorter growing season.

Are organic foods 100% free of glyphosphate?

No. A small amount of glyphosphate can get onto organic food by wind drift and animal manure.[40]

However, organic foods tend to have MUCH LOWER amounts of glyphosphate than nonorganic foods.

What does glyphophosphate do to plants?

Glyphosphate inhibits the shikimate pathway enzyme called EPSP synthase (EPSP-S). EPSP-S catalyzes a reaction where 2 PhosphoEnolPyruvates (PEP) and Shikimate 3-Phosphate are converted into 5-Enol-Pyruvyl-Shikimate-3-Phosphate (EPSP).

The EPSP can then be made into the aromatic amino acids phenyl-alanine, tyrosine, and tryptophan. These amino acid are used to make the neurotransmitters dopamine, epinephrine, serotonin, and melatonin, and thyroid hormone.[41]

Do companies sometimes cheat on organic?

---

37 "Toxic Legacy" by Stephanie Seneff, copyright 2021, page 11.
38   Toxic Legacy" by Stephanie Seneff, copyright 2021.
39 "Toxic Legacy" by Stephanie Seneff, copyright 2021.
40   "Glyphosphate rich air samples induce IL-33, TSLP and generate IL-13 dependent airway inflammation" Toxicology 0 (2014): 42-51, Sudhir Kumar et al.
41   "Toxic Legacy" by Stephanie Seneff, copyright 2021.

Sometimes they do. Usually they do not.

Some countries follow the rules more closely than others.

Some countries – like China – have so much pollution, that it is difficult for them to meet the standards of producing organic food, according to Mike Adams author of the book "Food Forensics" about food contaminants.

Do organic foods contain more nutrients than nonorganic?

That is a complex question.

Overall, it seems that the organic foods tend to be slightly more nutritious.

However, the main benefit of eating organic is to minimize exposure to herbicides and pesticides.

What is the proof that organic is better?

People who eat organic have much less herbicide and pesticide residues in their blood and urine.[42] [43]

People who eat organic have a lower risk of cancer.[44]

What's the deal with organic food and Russia?

Putin is hoping that Russia will become a leader in organic foods.[45]

When I was growing up in the 1970's and 1980's, Russia was considered a godless, commie, sh_thole. The only thing we admired about Russia was their wrestlers, and weightlifters – who we felt had an unfair advantage, because they were professionals, while our guys were true amateurs. Russia was famous for famine, and making excuses about "bad weather."

The fact that Russia now claims to have better soil quality is sad.

If we are at a restaurant, how can we minimize our exposure to herbicides, pesticides, and MSG?

Only eat plant foods, but avoid corn, soy, and other likely g-m-o foods.

For what plant foods is it especially important to eat organic?

Strawberries, because their shape is too difficult to wash.

Celery, perhaps because of the ridges.

Grapes because their skin is so thin, and too difficult to wash.

Spinach, because it's an above ground "leaf," and the nonorganic form tends to get sprayed too much.

The Environmental Working Group website – EWG dot org – has a "dirty dozen" list of plant foods for which it is especially recommended to only eat organic.

What about the clean 15 foods recommended by the EWG dot org?

42 "Excretion of herbicide glyphosate in older adults between 1993-2016" Jama 318, no 16(2017). Paul Mills et al.
43 "Detection of glyphosphate residues in animals and humans" journal of environmental and analytical toxicology 4 (2014): 210, Monika Kruger et al.
44 "Association of frequency of organic food consumption with cancer risk: Nutri Net Sante Prospective Study" Jama Intern Med 2018, Touvier et al.
45 "Putin wants Russia to become a world leader in organic food" Farmer's weekly, Dec 4, 2015, Phillip Case.

EWG says that there are 15 foods especially low in pesticides and herbicides which includes sweet peas, sweet potatos, and cabbage.

Foods that grow underground, like sweet potatos, tend to be less sprayed with pesticides.

What about cadmium?

Nonorganic foods tend to contain more cadmium. Cadmium is a heavy metal toxin.

What are the disadvantages of eating organic?

Costs a little bit more.

However, starch is cheap. A starch based organic diet is reasonably priced.

Fruit is more expensive.

What about the environment?

Organic is better for the environment. Nonorganic pollutes the soil, and waterways, and food, with herbicide, and pesticide residues.

What animals are fed with gmo crops?

Cows, chickens, pigs.

What foods have a gmo version?

Corn, soy, tomatos, cotton, papaya, canola, sugar beets, alfalfa. Also tobacco.

Are gmo's safe?

The risks are not yet clear. GMO's are sprayed with glyphosphate which is the reason I would NEVER eat gmo food. There are some scientists who are quite concerned about the risks of gmo.[46] [47] [48]

What's the significance of GMO soy?

I would not eat it.

GMO soy is used to provide protein for processed foods.

Do you ever eat soy?

No. Soy is a very complicated food. Soy can be processed in multiple ways.

In my opinion – soy – is too complicated. Although some nutrition experts claim that soy has potential benefits, none of them seem to outweigh the downsides; so I would never eat it.

Some authors say that soy is goitrogenic. Some authors write that some forms of soy are processed with hexane solvents. The amino acid composition of soy protein is unusual for a plant, and is associated with increasing insulin like growth factor (ILGF). Soy has very, very, high levels of estrogenic chemicals.

GMO soy is likely sprayed with glyphosphate. The majority of soy is gmo soy.

What's the bottom line on organic?

46 "Risk assessment of genetically modified crops for nutrition and health." Nutr Rev, 2009; 67:1-16. Calderon de la Barca et al.

47 "Toxic Legacy" a book written in 2021 by Stephanie Seneff, PhD about glyphosphate.

48 "Food Forensics: the hidden toxins lurking in your food, and how you can avoid them for lifelong health" by Mke Adams

I recommend that you ONLY EAT ORGANIC

because the herbicides and pesticides in nonorganic foods appear to have significant side effects, that can ruin your health, and be irreversible.

I NEVER eat nonorganic, other than on RARE occasions – like special events – where I might have to eat a little bit. Given that I never get invited anywhere, it's easy to avoid nonorganic food.

Chapter 9

Are Coffee and tea good for you?

Skeptical Reader (SR): Are coffee and tea good for you?

Vegan Prophet (VP): Rule #1 of "science:

> "He who pays the piper, calls the tune." - anonymous.

Whoever pays for research, controls the results.

Regular people are too poor to pay for anything. Therefore any food item that is a big money maker will have lots of "*research*," saying it's good.

"If you want to inspire confidence, give plenty of statistics. It does not matter that they should be accurate, or even intelligible, as long as there is enough of them." - Lewis Carroll, English author, (1832-1898).

Plant man Prometheus (Pmp): Rule #2 of "science."

> "When big money talks, the truth is shuts up." - anonymous.

Big money uses "information flooding" to dominate the debate.

I've gone to bookstores and looked at all the nutrition, and health books. There are 99 blatantly false books, for each true book.

On the internet, there are 99 nonsense promoters of MOFFUC'S PP items for each health vegan.

I have talked to thousands of people about nutrition. 99% think that coffee, tea, chicken, fish, fish oil, olive oil, and wine are "health foods."

The average person is easily fooled by bogus "science," which is just advertising.

SR: Will you stop it with all that theoretical bullshit. I asked a simple question. Are coffee and tea good for you?

VP: The reason for that preamble is help you to see through all the internet puff pieces, that recommend coffee and tea.

Silicone Man (SM): Most doctors and scientists drink coffee and tea. Are you saying they are ignorant?

Pmp: Yes. Most doctors and scientists don't know anything about nutrition. Most of them are conformists. They just copy what they see older doctors, and scientists doing.

Rip van Winkle: Medical and scientific training programs use the young people to do all the night shift work. The young people drink coffee to stay awake, and they become addicted.

SR: Is coffee and tea good for you? Yes or no?

VP: Coffee and tea both contain caffeine. Caffeine is a stress equivalent. Caffeine increases the same hormones as stress: cortisol and catecholamines.

Pmp: When someone says "I'm so stressed out, I need a cup of coffee," that indicates they have a low nutrition IQ.

VP: Cortisol increases blood glucose. Cortisol therefore increases insulin resistance. Increased insulin resistance means increased risk of diabetes.

Pmp: Cortisol suppresses the immune system. Immune suppression puts you at increased risk for infection.

Catecholamines can function as siderophores, to transfer iron to bacteria; which increases risk of infection.

VP: Cortisol is associated with insomnia. Insomnia is associated with sleep deprivation. Sleep deprivation is a stress equivalent; caffeine leads to a vicious cycle of poor sleep, and suboptimal health.

Rvw: Cortisol is associated with obesity, and with muscle wasting; increasing the risk of becoming fat and weak.

Pmp: Cortisol and catecholamines elevate blood pressure. Hypertension is associated with increased risk of atherosclerosis, impotence, myocardial infarction, and stroke.

Rvw: Catecholamines increase heart rate which can increase the risk of atrial fibrillation in vulnerable persons.

VP: Cortisol and catecholamines cause the blood to become more hypercoaguable by elevating fibrinogen, von Willenbrand factor, factor 8 (antihemophilic factor), and by increasing platelet activation.

According to some papers, increased platelet activation is associated with increased risk of metastatic cancer, because the activated platelets appear to shield metastatic cells from the immune system.

Pmp: Hypercoaguable blood is beneficial if a tiger scratches you. Hypercoaguable blood is not good if you are a modern sedentary person. Hypercoaguable blood puts you at increased risk for impotence, myocardial infarction, and stroke.

VP: Cortisol increases glutamate in the hippocampus, which can worsen hippocampal excitotoxicity, leading to anxiety, impaired memory, and neuronal cell death.

Rvw: Caffeine increases the risk of gastroesophageal reflux disease (GERD).

VP: Many people put milk in their coffee. Milk is associated with increased risk of prostate cancer, and lots of other diseases.

Pmp: Many people put sweeteners in their coffee which are not healthy.

SR: But what about tea? Tea tends to have less caffeine. Is tea good for you?

Rvw: Tea drinkers remind me of MJ smokers. They think they are clever, but they don't know what they are talking about.

VP: Tea concentrates aluminum. Aluminum is neurotoxic, and associated with increased risk of Alzheimer's disease.[49]

Pmp: Tea concentrates fluoride. Fluoride is associated with lowering of IQ.

SR: What about energy drinks?

---

49 "Imagine you are an aluminum atom" by Christopher Exley PhD, copyright 2020.

VP: Ha, ha, ha. Most energy drinks come in a can. A lot of cans are made out of aluminum.

Pmp: A lot of cans are lined with BPA, and potentially with some other estrogenic chemical. Some energy drinks contain MSG.

Rvw: If you are sleep deprived, or tired, and you have a long commute, then it might make sense to ingest a caffeinated beverage.

VP: To ingest caffeine on a routine basis is a detriment to your health.

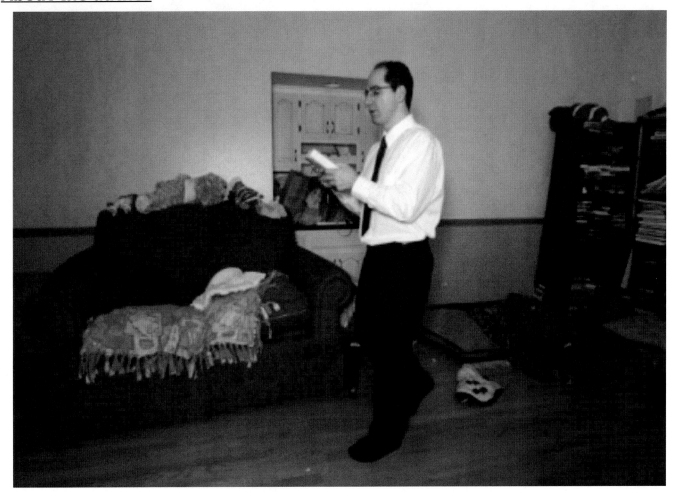

Fig 105: **Walking is a great exercise.** Author walking and reading. I often walk around the house while reading.

The book makes it more enjoyable.

I routinely walk while eating.

I often walk during conversation.

I go for a walk during study breaks.

Whenever taking a bathroom break, I try to walk to the farther bathroom, to get more exercise.

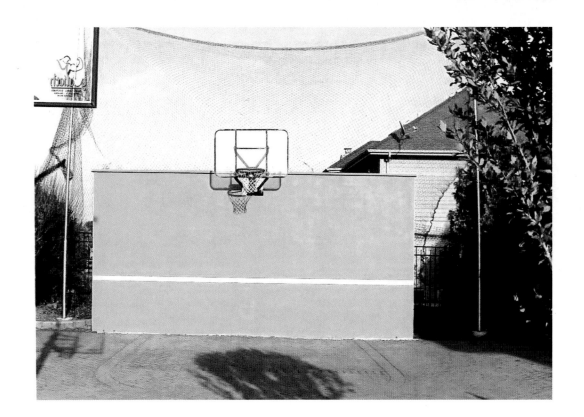

Fig 106: **At my old house, I had a tennis wall,** with an outdoor basketball hoop.

This provided great exercise and fun.

Everything was going great, until I pushed my luck.

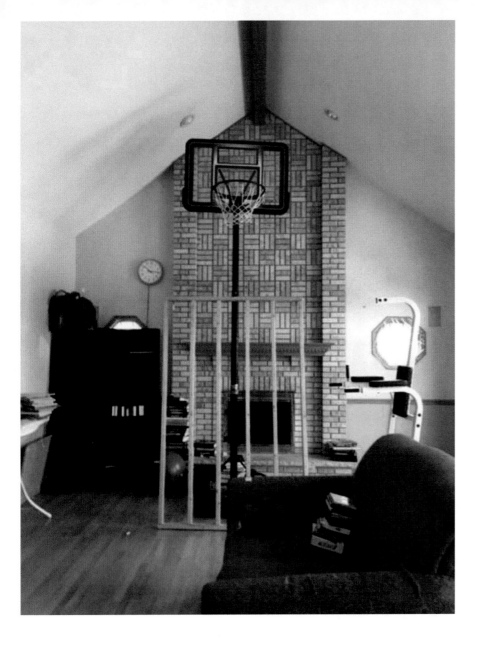

Fig 107: **Indoor basketball at my old house.** My son wanted to practice basketball.

He wanted to become a starter on the basketball team.

He said I was a bad parent, because I just worked all the time. He said that other dads helped their sons to get better at basketball.

Even though the old house already had a big outdoor pool, a big yard, and an indoor weight lifting room, wrestling room, and raquet ball court, I wanted more exercise.

When my wife was at work, my carpenter friend boarded up the windows, and we installed the portable basketball hoop. The room was already perfect, with a high ceiling and a wooden floor.

We loved indoor basketball.

Wife went ape shit bananas about it. Then she did her wicked witch imitation.

That's it! I'm sick of your crazy, autistic behavior. We are moving!

I'm going to buy a new house, and you're going to pay for it!

You have ruined the house. How can I have company over when the house looks like this?

I said that she should be happy to have such a unique house.

She said, all that dribbling is so noisy, it's driving me nuts! You are shaking the foundation of the house. You are lowering the property value.

This is a house, not a f_cking gymnasium!

She got so mad about it, that she went and bought a new house.

I had a choice: either join her in the new house = a wimpy, sissy, female sort of a house, with lots of flowers, but nowhere to exercise;

or to keep the old house, and get a divorce.

I wanted to keep the family together, so I sold the old house, and moved into the new house with her and the kids.

My basketball playing son said, "I can't believe you let mom control you like that. You are such a pussy. I have lost all respect for you."

I said, "I wanted to keep the family together. That's why I did it."

In retrospect:

I should've kept the old house. The kids would have wanted to move to the old house when they got older.

It would have meant divorce, but I'm tired of my wife bossing me around. Marriage gives too much power to the wife. Marriage puts the stupid person in charge of the smart person.

Girlfriends try harder, because they know it's easy for you to say goodbye to them, if they don't behave.

On the other hand:

It took a lot of time to maintain the old house. I had to do all the work, and pay all the bills.

The wife hated the old house, and refused to help with the management of it.

The new house is my wife's house. She does everything to maintain it.

That provides me with a lot of free time.

I lost my beloved old house, but gained a lot of free time.

That new free time is what makes it possible to write these books, and to make the you tube channel Peter Rogers MD.

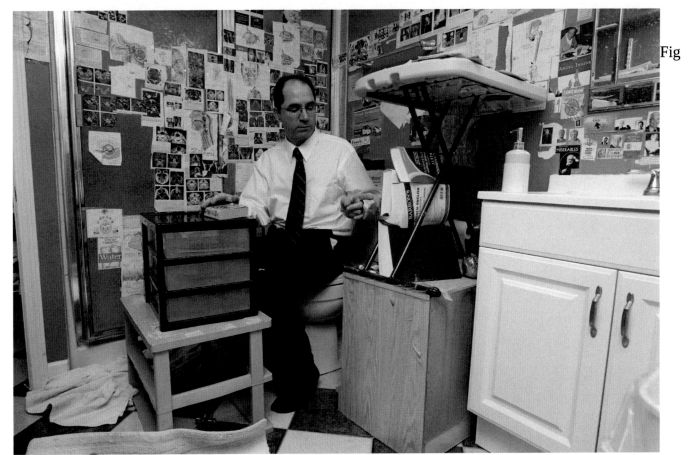

108: **The magic bathroom at the old house.** Great for reading. Usually had a hardcopy book on the portable table for #2's and a paper back on the other table for #1's.

I can't understand why my wife wasn't impressed by the magic bathroom. Of course, it was in the basement. She didn't want guests to know about it.

I showed it to every friend that ever visited. I got a perfect score on my neuroradiology boards, in large part from studying in the magic bathroom.

I had a Leitner box, flash card, spaced interval system on the far wall (not included in the picture).

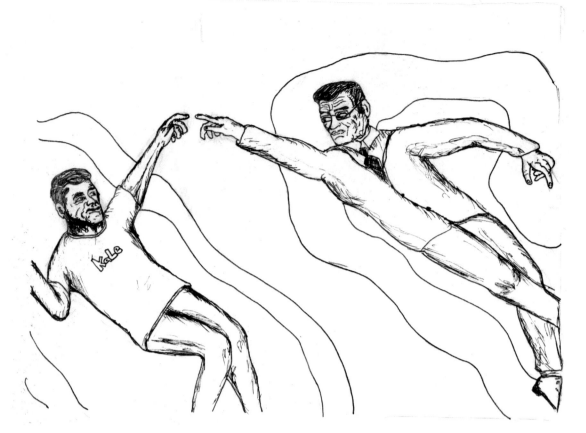

Fig 109: **Dr Caldwell Esselstyn speaks like the Old Testament God.**

No meat, not one bite!

No oil, not one drop!

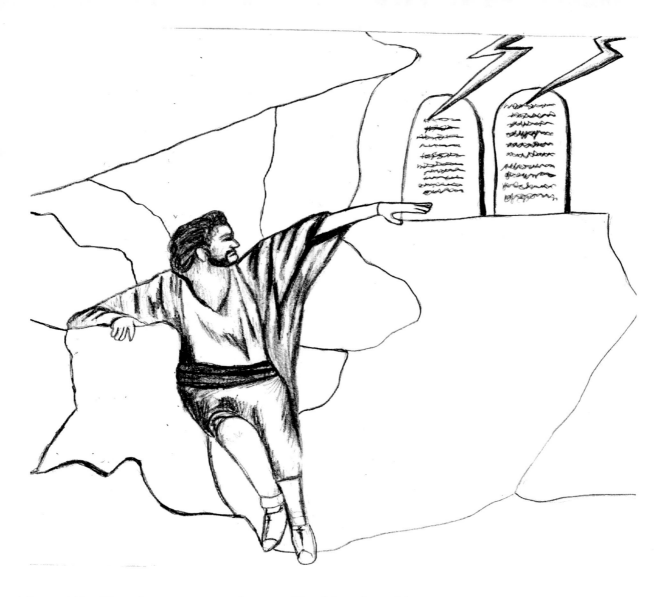

Figure 110: Obey the ten commandments of health and nutrition.

GO YE, AND TEACH all people,

in the name of the of the Starch, the Fruit, and the Vegetable.

BAPTIZE them with BEET juice,

and give them COMMUNION with a circular piece of POTATO.

Teach them to observe all things I have shown you:

and, behold, I am with you, always, even unto the end of the world.[50]

---

50 Parody of Matthew 28:19-20.

Notes:

Notes:

Notes:

Notes:

Made in the USA
Coppell, TX
05 December 2023

25339639R00102